ON THE LIST

Fixing America's Failing Organ Transplant System

STEVE FARBER
and HARLAN ABRAHAMS

RODALE

© 2009 by Harlan Abrahams and Steve Farber

Rodale books may be purchased for business or promotional use or for special sales. For information, please write to:
Special Markets Department, Rodale Inc., 733 Third Avenue, New York, NY 10017

Printed in the United States of America
Rodale Inc. makes every effort to use acid-free ♾, recycled paper ♻.

Book design by Christina Gaugler
Photographs on pages 111, 211, and 212 courtesy of the authors

Library of Congress Cataloging-in-Publication Data
Farber, Steve.
    On the list : fixing America's failing organ transplant system / Steve Farber and Harlan Abrahams.
        p.   cm.
    Includes bibliographical references.
    ISBN–13 978–1–60529–840–5 (hardcover)
    ISBN–10 1–60529–840–9 (hardcover)
    1. Transplantation of organs, tissues, etc.—United States.
I. Abrahams, Harlan.   II. Title.
RD120.7.F37   2009
617.9'54—dc22   2009001981

Distributed to the trade by Macmillan

2   4   6   8   10   9   7   5   3   1   hardcover

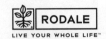

We inspire and enable people to improve their lives and the world around them
For more of our products visit **rodalestore.com** or call 800-848-4735

To Carolyn, Rachel, and Amelia, for their support,
and to Ernesto, for his courage
—Harlan

To my wife, Cindy, and my sons, Gregg, Brent, and Brad,
for their support, commitment, and courage;
and to my granddaughter, Andie,
to whom Gregg also gave the gift of life
—Steve

CONTENTS

PROLOGUE V

Part One: Lives in Jeopardy

Chapter One: A Tale of Two Transplants 3
Chapter Two: The Measles Cure 14
Chapter Three: Escape to a Better Life....................................... 23
Chapter Four: The Good Life, Threatened................................. 34
Chapter Five: Brotherly Love... 46

Part Two: A System in Distress

Chapter Six: The American Transplant System 61
Chapter Seven: The Global Markets for Organs........................ 73
Chapter Eight: Final Options 96
Chapter Nine: The Day of Our Surgeries.................................. 113
Chapter Ten: Fatally Flawed 127

Part Three: The Search for Solutions

Chapter Eleven: The Band-Aid Approach 151
Chapter Twelve: The Realities of Reform.................................. 177
Chapter Thirteen: A New Life and New Purpose...................... 201

EPILOGUE.. 213
AUTHORS' NOTE... 216
APPENDIX A: TRANSPLANT LAWS AROUND THE WORLD 217
APPENDIX B: NATIONAL ORGAN TRANSPLANT ACT 224
ENDNOTES... 240
ABOUT THE AUTHORS 272
INDEX... 274

PROLOGUE

My phones started ringing earlier than usual that morning. It was nearly May 2007 and I was used to phones ringing early in those days. My clients paid well, as always, and in return they expected constant access to me. I was also working hard to bring the Democratic National Convention to Denver in August 2008. My sons lived in New York, 2 hours ahead. People called early. But never that early.

"Hello," I answered, no doubt sounding cranky. I blinked at the digital clock on my nightstand.

"Have you heard? Have you heard!" demanded a voice both foggy and familiar.

Instant relief: It wasn't one of my sons. No family emergencies.

"Heard what?"

The voice spoke only a few short sentences. But, second by second, my jaw dropped lower and lower and my mouth sagged farther open. I hung up without even saying good-bye.

My wife, Cindy, turned away from me, muttering over the interruption. "What's wrong?" she slurred, still mostly asleep.

"Nothing," I said. Then I got out of bed, put on my robe, and rushed downstairs to my home office to boot up my computer. I read every English account of the event[1] that had awakened me so early that morning. The accounts were not entirely consistent, but they agreed on enough details to let my imagination fill in the rest.

April 27, 2007: On a winding back street on the Asian side of Istanbul, a small medical clinic hides behind the crumbling façade of a tenement. There must be at least two operating theaters, not state-of-the-art, perhaps, but adequate. Recovery areas for at least eight people occupy the second floor. There are hospital rooms, nurses' stations, all the necessary components. The place is neat, tidy, and scrubbed antiseptically clean.

Today a team of roughly 15 has just completed two kidney transplants behind the crumbing walls. In one, an Israeli Arab has donated to a South African in his sixties. In the other, a second Israeli Arab has donated to an Israeli Jew. The two transplants were performed nearly simultaneously by a Turkish surgeon assisted by Zaki Shapira, MD, the famous Israeli organ outlaw. Dr. Shapira, a pioneer in organ transplantation, often had been accused of brokering the illegal sale of organs, and his clinic was operating in contempt of a shutdown order issued a month before by a Turkish court for lacking a license to perform organ transplants. At 71, Dr. Shapira was too old to perform the illicit surgeries himself. But he was always right there in the operating theater, supervising in his green surgical scrubs and his purple knit cap.

The two donors and the two recipients are transferred to the recovery ward on the second floor of the little clinic. They are starting to come out of their surgical comas.

Two bursts of gunfire hasten the process.

The gunfire echoes through the hallways and up the stairs. It sounds like it's coming from the entryway to the clinic, where four gunmen have burst onto the scene. One of the transplant patients—let's call him Number One—hears it all too clearly, while two others swoon in delirium and the fourth languishes under anesthesia.

The bursts of gunfire are rapid: *rat-tat-tat*. There must be at least two semiautomatics, perhaps a Kalashnikov, perhaps an Uzi. And handguns, maybe a Stechkin or Makarov, maybe a rusty old Colt .45-caliber revolver. Whatever their make, they are wielded by four very angry men with black knit ski masks pulled over their faces.

The men are there to rob the clinic of its take for the day. They know all about the clinic because they are disgruntled past donors. Two claim never to have been paid; one claims never to have received the promised follow-up care; one simply regrets his decision to sell his kidney in the first place. They wave their guns and fire into the air.

An alternate version has Dr. Shapira stumbling upon the four robbers rifling through his personal belongings in his locker room, looking for the loot. Whatever the specifics, more gunshots are fired and the police are quickly summoned. They arrive in an instant, their sirens wailing and blue lights flashing.

A spectacular gun battle erupts. At least one policeman is shot.

Number One listens to the *rat-tat-tat*'s and *boom-boom-boom*'s exploding below. He hears screams from more than one person. There are, after all, other patients down there waiting for surgery. And he hears shouts, all in foreign languages. It's disconcerting. It's terrifying. And he can't do a thing about it because he is immobile from the surgery, lying beneath a web of tubes and sensors and monitors that are connected to his sedated body . . . to say nothing of the 8 inches of fresh sutures holding him closed.

Number One wonders if he'll be arrested. He wonders, indeed, if he'll survive.

Finally the shots, screams, and shouts die down. Orders are barked in Turkish. Heavy steps stomp up the stairs. Just like something out of the movie *Midnight Express*, the police are coming for him. Will he rot in a Turkish prison? Might he even die there?

I could have been Number One. I came within weeks of going to Turkey to buy a kidney I badly needed. My date with Dr. Zaki Shapira had been scheduled for May 16, 2004, almost exactly 3 years before this dramatic gun battle. This is my story. I was extremely lucky. I had a healthy, loving son who demanded that I accept his donation of a kidney. He knew I could not get that *Midnight Express* scenario out of my mind. So he saved me from running the risk of being Number One.

This is also the story of a courageous young Guatemalan immigrant named Ernesto Delaroca who donated his kidney to his sister on the same day and at the same hospital where I received the gift of life. Some who have seen us together have called us the peasant and the power broker, but I think of Ernesto as a hero.

Finally, this is a story of a world of ethics and medicine and law gone mad. It is a story of the dramatic shortage of transplant organs in America and throughout the world, a story of the growth of illicit organ markets in poor Third World countries, and the story of the failure of our legal, medical, and political establishments to deal with the problems.

Each year, 6,500 people die in America while waiting for organ transplants. That's more than twice the number of people we lost on September 11, 2001. And many of their deaths could be prevented. Our broken system of organ transplant policies and procedures needs fixing. It is both antiquated and ineffective. That's why I jumped at the chance to work with Harlan Abrahams when he approached me, 5 months after my surgery, with the idea of collaborating on a book that would weave my story together with Ernesto's and a deeper analysis of the crisis in organ transplant policy in America.

Harlan had been a partner at my law firm before he returned to a life of teaching and writing. He had been following the growth in the markets for human transplant organs for more than a decade. Together, we found we had a lot to say. We hope this book will help grease the wheels of change.

PART ONE

LIVES IN JEOPARDY

CHAPTER ONE

A TALE OF TWO TRANSPLANTS

On May 11, 2004, surgical nurses in green scrubs wheeled my oldest son, Gregg, from the operating room while they finished transplanting his kidney into me. Then they wheeled me out, cleaned the room, prepped for the next surgery, and wheeled in two Guatemalan immigrants, Ernesto Delaroca and his younger sister, Sandra.

The Farber and Delaroca families had converged in the same hospital that morning. We shared the same doctor, the same operating theater, and even the same waiting room.

But there the similarities stopped. Our separate journeys to the same destination illustrate the dramas and challenges faced by the many thousands whose lives depend on organ transplants at a time when there is a dramatic shortage of organs available to them.

My journey followed a road lined with intense family debate. We argued pros and cons. We argued most about the risks to his own health Gregg would face were he to donate his kidney to me. Why should he have to face those risks? I was 60, white, and wealthy. I shared the helm at the most politically powerful law firm in Colorado. Still, all that money and power could not erase the simple fact: Without a healthy kidney, I would soon die. What the wealth did give me were options that many others did not have.

Sandra, for example, could never have traveled across the globe to purchase a new kidney even though she too faced death without one. Fortunately, she had Ernesto. He was a family man and a hard worker. He had no money or power, but he had exactly what his sister needed: a healthy, compatible kidney. He freely gave his with little ado.

There's a certain irony to these stories. If the coda to my journey erupted in most dramatic fashion on the back streets of Istanbul 3 years after my surgery, then the prelude to Ernesto's journey began in equally dramatic fashion in 1984.

Back then, Cindy and I were preparing for Gregg's bar mitzvah the following year. We were so proud of him. He was handsome then, as he is now, big and smart and charming and articulate, a junior tennis star ranked first in his seven-state region. The theme of his bar mitzvah party would be Wimbledon. Steve Alvarez, Channel 7's senior sportscaster, would interview Gregg, and it would be projected on giant video screens for the 500 guests. There would be tables brimming with food, the abundance meant to evoke the athlete's limitless "training table." And there would be games and music so Denver's gentry could dance the night away. More would be spent on that party than most families in the world earn in years.

By the time Cindy and I were busy planning Gregg's big party, Ernesto, though less than a year older than Gregg, already had become a man. Born on April 10, 1973, in Guatemala City, he was a dark-skinned, boyish-faced youth with thick black hair, straight white teeth, and a well-muscled body. His parents, Valentine and Rosalea, made their home in a tiny one-room hovel in the city, a place divided by curtains into even tinier rooms. They worked the fields outside of town.

Valentine worked especially hard and bought 2 acres of good land, then bought a few more acres, until he finally owned 11 acres in the countryside between the city and the village of Aldea, 40 miles away, where Rosalea's sister and her family lived.

Ernesto loved his parents. His mother had black hair so long that she tied it in a braid that fell all the way to her knees. She was a great cook. His favorite dish was her *carne guisada*—beef and rice with tomato—though today he favors pasta with shrimp. His father was tall and skinny, a *campesino*, a peasant, who farmed beans, corn, and rice.

Valentine sometimes took Ernesto fishing, but they didn't have money for treats. Ernesto's best memories of Valentine were taking the bus with him from the outskirts of the city to the family fields to spend the day working together under the sun. That way the son had his father all to himself. They could work side by side in peace.

The family barely got by. They had no telephone or television, but they did have an old radio. Ernesto recalls hearing a lot of talk and not much music on that old radio.

Guatemala was a troubled country back then, torn by insurgency and civil war from the early 1960s until a formal peace agreement was signed in 1996. Communists had taken Cuba and were crawling all over Latin America, fomenting violent revolution. The United States supported anyone, however awful, who stood against the commies.

In March 1982, shortly after presidential elections were held in Guatemala, General José Efraín Ríos Montt, an evangelical born-again Christian, seized power in a coup backed by the CIA and the Reagan administration.[1] A devout anticommunist, Ríos Montt's relations with the United States spanned decades and included several presidential administrations, the CIA, the Pentagon's School of the Americas—the infamous "coup school"—and the religious right. He blamed Guatemala's Catholic priests for his defeat in the 1974 presidential elections. The priests had championed the country's poor Mayan peasants, its indigenous underclass who desired land and other reforms, and had leaned neither left not right. Ríos Montt had claimed the priests were leftist agents and agitators. In 1978, he left the Catholic Church and became a minister in the Church of the World, based in California. He used to call Jerry Falwell and Pat Robertson his friends.

Yet, when measured by his actions, Ríos Montt was no Christian. His years in power marked some of the bloodiest in the history of Central America. Efforts to bring "Guatemala's Pinochet" to justice on charges of genocide have repeatedly failed.

After seizing power in 1982, Ríos Montt launched a bloody reign of terror against those he labeled "insurgents and dissidents"— mostly anyone who disagreed with his autocratic ways. Kidnappings, torture, extrajudicial assassinations, and secret military tribunals rained horror upon the people. A state of siege was declared.

The campaign known as *frijoles y fusiles*—beans and guns— represented the tyrant's effort to subdue the indigenous Mayan population, many of whom were included in the dictator's definition of "insurgents and dissidents." This campaign featured a scorched-earth policy patterned on those used by the French in Algiers and the United States in Vietnam. Entire villages were annihilated, razed, wiped from the face of the earth.[2] Thousands of people were killed or disappeared during the 18-month rule of Ríos Montt. Amnesty International reports that 2,600 indigent Guatemalans and peasant farmers died in extrajudicial killings during the March-to-July period alone: "People of all ages were not only shot, they were burned alive, hacked to death, disemboweled, drowned, beheaded. Small children were smashed against rocks or bayoneted to death."[3]

On August 8, 1983, General Oscar Humberto Mejía Victores staged another coup and ousted Ríos Montt from power. Unfortunately, this general was even more authoritarian and repressive than his predecessor. The killings continued.

At about 4:00 a.m. on an ordinary day in 1984, a dozen gunmen burst into the Delarocas' one-room home. They weren't wearing helmets, caps, or masks, but they did wear the green uniforms of soldiers and they carried soldiers' rifles. Valentine and Rosalea were sleeping on one side of the curtain while Ernesto, 11, slept on the other side with his sister, Sandra, then a tiny baby, and his brother, Edgar, who was 2 years old.

Ernesto saw the flimsy curtain ripped aside. Before he could move, one of the soldiers shouted at him, *"¡Quedate callado!"*—Stay quiet!

Another snapped, *"¡Note mueves!"*—Don't move!

Ernesto was frozen, his eyes wide with fear.

Half the soldiers dragged Valentine and Rosalea from the room. That was the last Ernesto saw of them. The rest of the soldiers stayed behind for about 45 minutes. Ernesto didn't move. He didn't speak. He didn't even cry.

Sandra and Edgar didn't cause any trouble.

There was no screaming. There were no gunshots. All was quiet.

Ernesto's parents simply disappeared.

When the soldiers who had stayed behind finally left, Ernesto didn't wait for tears or panic. He knew they could come back at any moment. So he gathered a few things and, carrying little Sandra, led Edgar out of their one-room home, never to return. He took them to the bus stop and waited for the old bus that went to the fields.

Then Ernesto Delaroca got on that bus with his infant sister and his toddler brother and took them past his father's fields, all the way to Aldea, where his mother's sister lived with her husband and their children. When Ernesto told his aunt what had happened, they cried in each other's arms. Finally, there was time for tears.

Ernesto and his family never found out what happened to Valentine and Rosalea. The family never talked about their disappearance.

Later, when Ernesto grew older and tried to make inquiries, no one in the government would acknowledge knowing anything. "They gave me the runaround," he says, sadly shaking his head.

When asked if his parents were "political," Ernesto emphatically says, "No." Although the shape of his eyes might suggest otherwise, he also claims his family has no Indian blood. Besides, the terror of the right-wing death squads knew no strict racial boundaries. Peasant farmers were targeted as often as the indigenous Mayans.

And so another disappearance has never been explained.

When asked if he still thinks about that night in 1984, Ernesto says, "Not often." He made peace with it long ago. He's happy with his life. Every once in a while someone in his family says his parents might still be alive. Someday they might show up.

But Ernesto knows it's not true. He smiles and shakes his head. He knows what happened to his parents that night. That night was the first time he saved Sandra's life.

My story and Ernesto's story are part of a bigger story. This is the saga of the shortage of transplant organs throughout the world and the rise of markets that defy the taboos to supply the demand. These markets lie at the intersection of three great forces that drive today's events: economic forces like globalization that spread capitalism to Third World countries, political forces like sovereignty that demand respect for the boundaries of nations, and legal forces like constitutionalism that impose the rule of law.

US law creates a complex system for allocating transplant organs, a system torn between factors skewed toward geography and those skewed toward need. Geography tends to favor rural states while need tends to favor urban areas.[4] Federal and state laws prohibit the buying and selling of organs for transplantation and therapy; these laws preclude the development of an American market to deal with the resulting shortages.[5]

That's right. The buying and selling of human organs for purposes other than transplantation and therapy are allowed.[6] For example, organs may be bought and sold—and commonly are—for research and educational purposes.

But not to save a person's life! This apparent inconsistency arises most often with postmortem donations,[7] also called cadaveric donations. But other, thornier issues arise in the context of live organ donation, usually because the risks to the donor's health must be weighed against the needs of the recipient. And, since kidneys are organs that come in pairs and only one is needed to live, the issues of live organ donation arise most frequently in cases of kidney transplants.

The United Network for Organ Sharing (UNOS), a nonprofit organization based in Richmond, Virginia, administers America's only Organ Procurement and Transplantation Network (OPTN), created by Congress in 1984.[8] UNOS reports that the waiting list for kidneys topped 60,000 for the first time in October 2004. More than 75 percent of the 99,000 patients on the waiting list as of May 22, 2008, have kidney disease. More than 6,500—twice the number lost in the 9/11 attacks—die each year while waiting for kidneys and other organs.[9]

Many of these deaths could be prevented. Yet the lists are long, the wait is long, the issues are so very complex. The system is paralyzed. Unless you have a good match in a friend or relative who will give you a kidney, your chance of being among the doomed is too high for comfort.

When faced with death, people seek solutions. In a world of globalized markets and capitalism triumphant, it doesn't take rocket science to ask: With so many unnecessary deaths and such drastic shortages, why not stimulate the supply of kidneys by allowing their purchase and sale?

A few years ago the idea sounded preposterous, but today . . . well, things change.

Fifteen years ago the idea of creating functioning capitalist markets for human transplant organs was little more than futuristic fantasy. Today, writes Debra Satz of Stanford University, "There is a growing, well-documented black market in organs like corneas and lobes of livers and especially kidneys."[10]

Web sites crowding the Internet extol the utility, compassion, and workability of free markets for human transplant organs. Yet only in Iran[11] is there a fully legalized and fully regulated market for organs—with countries like Pakistan and the Philippines close behind in allowing the sale of kidneys from private parties. The organ markets in most of the rest of the world, in countries like Turkey and India and South Africa, may be called "black," but in reality they lurk between black and gray. They fall through the cracks of legality.

These cracks are created by the collision of the three great forces that drive today's events. Business in the 21st century is globalized. Markets know no national boundaries. Multinational companies operate internationally, and the maze of differing and conflicting rules is astounding. Yet that is what happens when capitalism triumphs.

And when capitalism triumphs, things both tangible and intangible become not merely commodities, but "commodified."[12] Today's goods and services are being chopped into specialties, standardized, branded, packaged, franchised, rendered impersonal. Intellectual property reduces to shrink-wrap. Human organs— precious things of immeasurable value—become commodities to be bought and sold.

That is, in fact, exactly what the champions of the free market approach advocate. Call them the Free Market Camp. They insist, "Let the market work it out. The problem will solve itself if you legalize the buying and selling of organs. The greatest good for the greatest number will be achieved through the efficiencies of supply and demand."

At the same time, equally forceful arguments are made against the buying and selling of organs—making flesh into commodity—by human rights activists.[13] Call them the Human Rights Camp. "*Noooo!*" scream their Web sites, "the free market cannot be trusted to work it out! It's immoral and unethical and it exploits the poor. We should not allow payments to donors, period." Is there no other way?

We can buy and sell blood and semen and eggs. We can rent a woman's uterus. We can even buy and sell organs for purposes other than therapy and transplantation. Perhaps there is a middle ground between prohibition and unbridled market freedom.

While academics, theorists, and moralists debate, real markets for organs are growing in developing countries. And Americans can do little about these markets. We project democratic values and respect for sovereignty and usually avoid involving ourselves in the internal affairs of other nations.

Indeed, the politics of sovereignty reinforces the demands of globalization when it comes to organ markets. Sovereignty connotes an absolutist idea that governments can do whatever they want inside their own borders. This connotation emphasizes territorial rigidity and a focus on the nation-state. In reality, however, sovereignty is a flexible, relative concept. The attributes of sovereignty—an identifiable population living inside identifiable borders *plus* a government that controls that population within those borders *plus* broad international recognition—appear in a variety of mixtures.[14] Borders change. Populations migrate. Governments fall. Some nation-states become failed states.

What's more, the forces of economics and globalization predictably collide with the forces of politics and sovereignty. Transnational intergovernmental organizations like the International Monetary Fund, the World Trade Organization, and the United Nations transcend their nation-state members, often imposing their will on the weaker ones. Globalized nongovernmental organizations like Greenpeace and Amnesty International challenge the functions and functioning of nation-states. Terrorist groups like al-Qaeda wage asymmetric war against nations and cultures.

Still, it's not as if nations with borders have disappeared. Rather, the players on the international chessboard have increased in number, character, and density. And to make matters more complex, the rule of law intersects and collides with the forces of globalization and sovereignty. A vast number of laws and regulations address and resolve the conflicts between economics and politics that arise in our affairs.

None of these forces is all-powerful. Each depends upon the dispersal of power. Capitalism depends upon having a lot of buyers and sellers acting in the marketplace. Democracy depends upon having a people to govern themselves. And constitutionalism depends upon powers being fragmented into different branches of government, with checks and balances limiting that government's reach and authority.

So globalization creates the spread of markets. Capitalism rationalizes the process by which organs become commodities. Sovereignty limits our government's ability to interfere in the internal affairs of other countries, insulating organ markets where they exist. And the bewildering array of inconsistent laws, rules, and customs throughout the world provides cover for the buyers, sellers, and brokers of organs.

My story touches upon some of these issues. Ernesto's story touches upon others. Together our stories demonstrate why we need major organ transplant reform in America. We simply have to address the drastic shortage of organs we face here at home.

CHAPTER TWO

THE MEASLES CURE

The phone call came from nearly 60 years in my past. A retired nurse in her eighties phoned my office and asked if I was "the same Steve Farber" who had been a patient at Children's Hospital back in 1946. It was a jarring moment. Though I am well known in my community, few people are aware of that phase of my life.

Still, this old woman claimed that she had cared for me and because my case was so compelling, she had never forgotten my name. After seeing and hearing of me often in the Denver news, she finally decided to see if I was the same boy whose life she had helped to save with a most unusual treatment.

Intrigued by her call, I invited this woman to lunch. We both ordered salads. She told me about the day my mother had brought her "fat" little baby to the hospital. Her recollections merged with my family's mythology. She filled in some fine detail.

I was 18 months old when my parents took me to the Mayo Clinic in Rochester, Minnesota. I was born in September 1943, so it must have been early 1946. My father, Nathan—everyone called him Nate—ran a fruit stand in the old Loop Market near the Central Bank Building. It was called the Loop Market because it was where the streetcars made their loop to turn around. The draft exempted food producers, so my father didn't have to go to war. My mother, Janet, worked sales at the May Company department store. We were lower-middle-class Jews living on the west side of Denver.

My parents took me to the Mayo Clinic because I was urinating blood. I had suffered strep throat, and in those days strep throat often went undetected and untreated. And if you didn't detect it or treat it, it could lead to rheumatic fever or kidney damage. In my case it led to kidney damage. The doctors at Mayo told my parents that my kidneys "had turned to stone." They were not functioning. They were terribly damaged.

My parents were also told that I probably would not survive. They were told to go back home and wait. When they begged to know if there was anything at all that could be done for me, they were told to take me back to Children's Hospital in Denver and have them expose me to measles or some other disease that causes high fevers.

Why measles? Because tests had shown that sometimes a high fever could get kidneys working again—"shocking" them into functioning—and even reversing the damage. Decades later, I questioned my doctors about this treatment: Had they ever heard of it? Is this treatment still used? Isn't it dangerous? Most simply shrugged and said they either hadn't heard of it or there really weren't any studies about it. They never questioned the anecdotal results that prompted the treatment, however.

So my parents returned to Denver and my mother took me to Children's Hospital. She was only 23 at the time and it was a terrible ordeal for her. It was very hard on my father, too. He started drinking heavily as my condition worsened.

By the time my mother handed me over to the nurses at Children's Hospital, I was starting to get fat, a sure sign that my kidneys were failing and my body was retaining fluids. My mother was desperate.

She said to the nurses, "The doctors all say my boy will probably die, so I'm turning him over to you. Do whatever you can to make him live, because no one else thinks he will."

So they put me in the measles ward. My earliest recollections from childhood go back to that place. I swear I can remember it: the stark and sterile rooms and hallways, and my feelings of fear and abandonment when my parents left me there. Though I can't recall the faces of the nurses or other kids who were there, the look and feel of the place haunt me to this day. It was a place full of loneliness and fear and the sounds of sick kids crying through the night.

But at first I didn't catch the measles. My stay grew from days into weeks—longer than anyone had expected. Then the nurses made me eat food the sick kids had chewed so I would get their measles! And finally I did catch the disease—"rubeola," according to my records. And the virus did its job, driving up my temperature and somehow jump-starting my kidneys.

It was a miracle. I lived. My father promptly gave up his drinking. I think he must have made a bargain with God: "Let my son live and I'll live a clean life."

Things went back to normal. But I still had to have checkups once every month. I got a lot of shots and I had to urinate for the doctors and they put needles up my penis. Let me tell you, it was no fun. Sometimes they would say there was too much albumin or protein in my urine and my kidneys weren't filtering enough. So then I had to get more shots and it was even less fun. Then I was 5 and I stopped having monthly checkups, though no one ever told me why. I assume the doctors thought I had finally grown out of the danger.

Today people ask me if I really remember all these things or were they simply told to me so many times that I think I remember them. After all, I was only 18 months old when this happened. Well, for some reason, I have always had detailed memories of this and most of the other important times in my life. I can close my eyes today and picture that measles ward at Children's Hospital.

In 1996, I traveled with Cindy and her mother to the same Mayo

Clinic for treatment of my mother-in-law's cancer. I looked through the darkened window of the stretch limousine that was taking us to Rochester and I had the most vivid memory of having been there before, even though I hadn't been back since my parents had taken me there as a toddler with bad kidneys. I remembered the steel gray sky and the tall gray buildings.

So for me, it's a real memory, not just a suggestion.

The "measles cure" may sound fanciful, maybe even radical, but in 1946 there weren't many options available to me or my doctors. The widespread use of dialysis to cleanse the blood of impurities through ultrafiltration was still a decade away. And while the idea of organ transplantation dates back to ancient Greek and Hindu mythology, modern transplant medicine didn't really get started until World War II.[1]

The Battle of Britain provided plenty of burned pilots for the plastic surgeons to work on. Sir Archibald McIndoe, MD, worked for the Royal Air Force in Sussex, treating deep burns and facial disfigurement. He did a lot of skin grafts. His staff called him the Maestro. He and others observed something over and over again: Skin from one part of a person's body would graft to another part of the body, but skin taken from one person would not permanently graft to the skin of another.

That's where Peter Medawar, MD, came in. He was asked by Britain's Medical Research Council to investigate the phenomenon. In hindsight it seems obvious: The body's immune system rejects the tissues or organs of another. After the war, Dr. Medawar continued his research, shifting his emphasis to efforts to suppress the immune system so the body could better tolerate tissue grafts. These efforts built on his earlier research into tissue culture and the regeneration of nerves by focusing on problems of pigmentation and skin grafting in cattle—in particular the differences between "fraternal" and "identical" twins in accepting or rejecting skin grafts. Dr. Medawar's experiments led him to conclude that "actively acquired tolerance" of skin grafts could be artificially reproduced. These efforts earned him the Nobel Prize in Physiology or Medicine in 1960 for his discovery of "acquired immunological tolerance."

And that was the beginning of one of the two major branches of modern transplant medicine. This branch searches for ways for one person to better accept the organs of another. The better the acceptance, the less suppression of the immune system is needed, and the fewer the side effects and dangers of transplantation. First these researchers developed cortisone, then azathioprine.

The next generation of researchers brought us Sir Roy Calne, MD, who in 1968 performed Europe's first liver transplant. Dr. Calne still sports a permanent twinkle behind his thick, goggle-eyed glasses. His bold, colorful paintings of transplant surgeries and patients have become legendary in both the medical world and the art world. He is the guy who developed cyclosporine and introduced it to clinical practice in 1978.

Cyclosporine was the first major immunosuppressant drug to be widely used after organ transplants to reduce the activity of the patient's immune system and so the risk of organ rejection. It was initially isolated from a Norwegian soil sample and contains D-amino acids, which are rarely encountered in nature.

With cyclosporine, the opportunities for the second branch of modern transplant medicine simply exploded. This is the surgical branch, incorporating the doctors and nurses in the operating room. They're the ones who wield the knives, while the doctors from the first branch prescribe the drugs. And the pioneers of this second branch are as fascinating as the pioneers of the first branch.

In the 3rd century, for example, saints Damian and Cosmas supposedly replaced the gangrenous leg of the Roman deacon Justinian with the healthy leg of a recently deceased Ethiopian. There's a 16th-century painting that shows the black leg being attached to the white body.

But the modern era of transplant surgery began in Boston in 1954 when another future Nobel Prize winner, Joseph Murray, MD, performed the first successful kidney transplant between male identical twins. The surgery worked because no suppression of the immune system was needed: The twins were genetically identical, so the recipient's body had no reason to reject the donor's organ.

A lung was transplanted from a deceased donor to a lung cancer patient as early as 1963 in Mississippi, but the man survived for only 18 days. In Denver, at the same hospital where I later received the gift of life, Thomas Starzl, MD, performed the first successful liver transplant in 1967.

And who can forget the media circus that surrounded the first heart transplant, performed in 1967 by Christiaan Barnard, MD, in South Africa? His patient died only 18 days later, like the lung recipient in Mississippi, but his second heart transplant patient lived for 19 whole months! Sensational but disappointing results like these would plague the transplant surgeons as they awaited each advance by drug researchers.

With the introduction of cyclosporine in 1973, the art and science of organ transplantation finally moved from experiment to treatment. That means the use of human organ transplants as a practical medical therapy is only 36 years old.

While Dr. Barnard was busy performing the first heart transplants, I was getting ready to graduate from law school at the University of Colorado. I remember seeing the headlines when he did it, but other matters were gobbling up the news. Men were going to the moon. The ghettos were in flames. The Vietnam War, civil rights, assassinations, and *Sgt. Pepper's Lonely Hearts Club Band* burst onto the American consciousness in real time.

I had grown up not thinking much about my illness as a toddler. Every once in a while one of my parents' friends or one of our relatives would refer to me, when supposedly out of earshot, as the "sick baby," but I really never thought much about it.

I just wanted to get outdoors and play sports like all the other kids. But my mom remembered my dark days in Children's Hospital all too clearly. She was probably too protective of me. Far too often she would say no.

Then my dad would have to intervene and say, "He's going to do it anyway, Janet, so go ahead and let him do it."

Finally I got to play sports. And my mom got to give me the lecture she gave me over and over again throughout my childhood: "From the time you were little, God gave you life for a purpose. It's up to you to figure out what that purpose is."

So I guess it must be my mother's fault that I have always had a strong sense of destiny or purpose. I always felt more spiritual than the other kids. I studied all the major religions—Judaism, Christianity, Islam, Hinduism, and Buddhism—and I don't mean to sound fatalistic about this, since I'm not really sure I believe in these things, but so many things—both good and bad—have just . . . happened to me. I felt I had to succeed because my mother had put the onus on me.

Eventually I grew strong and got really good at sports. At 16 I played basketball at summer camp with Bill Bradley, who later became a US senator. We're still friends today. I graduated high school and went to college, then law school at the University of Colorado at Boulder. Shortly after I graduated, I founded my law firm in Denver with two of my boyhood friends, Norm Brownstein and Jack Hyatt.

Jack was the intellectual. I'd served with him on the law review.

Norm was great with people. Together we moved from a scrappy general practice to a firm that specialized in real estate law at a time when real estate was booming in Colorado. Today we have more than 200 lawyers in Colorado, New Mexico, Nevada, California, and Washington, DC. We have departments that cover all the major branches of law.

As we built our firm, Norm and I both took an interest in politics. It started out as community service coupled with an intense desire to support the State of Israel. The land of the Jews, our kinfolk, had suffered from repeated Arab assaults. Israel needed every dollar of American aid it could get. We started lobbying for the cause.

Our interest in politics grew into a passion that soon melded with our business as lawyers. It's very symbiotic. Over the years we have hosted countless fund-raisers and gotten involved with political causes and candidates from both parties.

I get consulted frequently by politicians at both the state and federal levels. I was honored when former president Bill Clinton, in town to promote his memoir and library, chose to have a private lunch and signing at my home in southeast Denver.

As I became successful in law, business, politics, and lobbying, some people started to call me a power broker. I've never really liked the label, but I suppose it sticks. In 1998 the Denver magazine *5280* named me the most powerful man in Colorado, ahead of the governor and mayor of Denver. My head shot filled the cover, which caused me to feel a mixture of pride and embarrassment.

Five years later, the local columnist and radio talk show host Peter Boyles wrote: "Denver's most powerful lobbyists are courted not just locally but by governors and presidential hopefuls. Steve Farber and Norm Brownstein have come a long way from their humble beginnings."[2]

By late spring 2003, I was sitting on top of the world. I had wealth and influence in my community. My three sons were fully grown and strong and healthy. What more could I possibly want?

I was able to wield that influence of mine over so many things. What I could not do was influence what was happening inside my body. In fact, I didn't even know it was happening.

My history as a "sick boy" was catching up to me.

CHAPTER THREE

ESCAPE TO A BETTER LIFE

rnesto Delaroca did not come legally to the United States. He had no money in the pockets of his tattered jeans. He left a country where he had no political power to go to one where he would have none once again. But at least in America, he could pursue economic opportunities and there would be little danger of being dragged away by a death squad in the middle of the night.

From the ages of 11 to 22, Ernesto worked his aunt and uncle's fields in Aldea. They raised him, Sandra, and Edgar as their own children. No one ever talked about the disappearance of Valentine and Rosalea. No one dared to confirm whether the government had seized the 11 acres Valentine had accumulated over his years of hard work. After that first awful night when Ernesto had cried in the arms of his aunt Otilia, nothing more was said.

Ernesto kept it all bottled up inside. He would go through the cycles with everyone else. For 2 weeks they would plant their corn, beans, watermelons, and vegetables. He always loved his watermelons. They would tend their crops, weed them, and grow them. Then, 3 months later, they would harvest them and start all over again.

Ernesto went to school for only 3 years—grades three, four, and five. But he had always been smart, and he grew into a handsome young man, with his bright white teeth and wispy moustache and thick black hair. Finding girlfriends was never a problem.

His family had an old 1978 Toyota. It was battered and bruised from a life of driving up and down the rutted rural roads of Guatemala, picking up people to go pick cotton in the fields, then later dropping them off at the end of the day. That's how the peasants earned extra money. The car became Ernesto's. It had a radio and even a cassette player, and when he drove it, he played music on them all the time.

By 1995, Otilia's son Oswaldo was working a construction job in Denver. He had been in the United States for 10 years. Before he came to America, he had been like a big brother to Ernesto. One day he called Ernesto on the phone and they talked.

"How's it working?" asked Ernesto.

"I am working very hard," answered Oswaldo, "but I can go anywhere I want. It's wonderful. I would very much like for you to come here and work with me."

Ernesto immediately accepted Oswaldo's invitation. Now 22 years old, he traveled to Mexico's border with Texas near El Paso. For most of the way, he flew with about 30 other people in a small, propeller-driven airplane. The man who operated the air service also taught his passengers how to cross the border without being detected—all for a fee, of course.

This was long before 9/11. The border was porous. There was no need for a visa. When asked how he got across, Ernesto makes his hand undulate like a wave of water.

He simply jumped with his 30 companions into the shallow waters of the Rio Grande and they quickly spread out over the river, as their guide had taught them. They spread so far apart, in fact, they could barely see each other. It was late in the afternoon of June 14 and it was "a little hot," as Ernesto recalls.

"But it was a piece of cake," he says, smiling and snapping his fingers. Soon he was living with Oswaldo and working as a dishwasher at a restaurant in Westminster.

Ernesto's smarts are practical. He learns quickly. He picked up English. In 6 months he was promoted from dishwasher to prep cook. He was still working there when, in May 1997, he heard that his aunt Otilia—who had raised him, Edgar, and Sandra as her own—had died at the age of 54 of bone cancer.

Ernesto and Oswaldo flew home to Guatemala for Otilia's funeral. It was still before 9/11. They needed neither passports nor visas. The only documents they needed to board their international flight were their national "certificates" or ID cards. Ernesto stayed in the little village of Aldea for 2 weeks after Otilia's funeral. That's when he met Gicela, his future wife. Two days after the funeral, she saw him shopping in the village. She approached him. "I'm sorry about your aunt," she said, introducing herself. "I saw you at the funeral, but I didn't get the chance to tell you then."

They began talking. And talking. And talking. Gicela became Ernesto's girlfriend.

Soon, however, he had to return to the United States. He and Oswaldo crossed the border the same way they had gone across the first time. "That's right," says Ernesto, making that waving-water motion with his hand. Again, no patrols and no trouble.

After he returned home to Denver, Ernesto began exchanging letters with Gicela. He called her every weekend on the telephone and they would talk for as long as he could afford. Their love grew in letters and phone calls over the next year.

In 1998 he returned to Aldea, this time to bring back Sandra, Edgar, and Gicela. Once again he gathered his little brother and his little sister to his side and took them to a new land. But this time he brought his fiancée as well. They rode on a rickety bus from Guatemala through Mexico, all the way to the border with Texas.

This time Ernesto needed no guidance. He taught Sandra, Edgar, and Gicela exactly what to do. "We all jumped into the river," says Ernesto. "It wasn't very deep. It came to above our ankles and below our knees." He points to his shins: "To here."

The four spread out, crossed the river, and found each other on the American side of the border near El Paso. They dried themselves off, walked into town, hopped on a Greyhound bus, and rode to Denver. Edgar went to work at the same restaurant in Westminster where Ernesto worked. At the time, Sandra and Gicela did not have jobs.

Ernesto knew it was time to "become legal." His family was back together and they needed to take the next step together. With his meager earnings, he hired an immigration lawyer named Richard Garcia and paid him $4,000 to make the family legal. It was a long process that required long hours of filling out Immigration and Naturalization Service forms and stretched from late 1998 into 2000.

"He's a big guy," says Ernesto of Garcia, "a really good guy."

Garcia told Ernesto he would have to marry Gicela to make her legal, as well. But they had no legitimate American identification papers, so they couldn't get married in Colorado, where they lived and worked. So they traveled to California, where they paid someone who knew someone in the Hispanic community, and they got married and acquired the papers to prove it. They returned and rented a house in Lakewood, just west of Denver and south of Westminster. They lived quiet lives and continued to work hard.

Ernesto calls himself a Christian. He doesn't drink or smoke. Nor does Gicela.

While Garcia, their lawyer, was working to get them "made legal," he naturally had to question them about their backgrounds and any claims they might have to stay inside the sovereign borders of the United States as political refugees rather than mere immigrants.

"Do you have any grounds for asylum?" asked the lawyer as a matter of course.

Having such grounds would hasten the process and ensure better results.

It didn't take long for Ernesto to call Gicela, Sandra, Edgar, and Richard Garcia together in the tiny living room of the family's home to talk about the question. They sat in a tight little circle on the carpet, speaking only in Spanish. And for the very first time, Ernesto told the story of how he, Sandra, and Edgar had come to live with their aunt Otilia and uncle José in Aldea after the right-wing death squad dragged off their real parents—Valentine and Roselea—in the dead of night.

Everyone sat stunned. No one moved and no one interrupted as Ernesto told them everything they needed to know to claim asylum as political refugees from Guatemala. When Ernesto finished, Garcia left him alone to face Edgar, Sandra, and Gicela.

Edgar immediately asked, "Is it all true?"

"Yes," Ernesto said sadly, "it's all true."

The living room fell silent. Shock waves rolled over the family as everyone processed the information Ernesto had disclosed.

Then Sandra started sobbing. She had always thought Otilia was her mother. Though she did not seem angry or confused, inside she was "freaking out," according to Ernesto.

After that fateful family discussion, which did pave the way for their asylum, Sandra began acting like a different person. She cried a lot, often for no apparent reason. She talked much less than before. She became quiet and withdrawn for long periods. And while she didn't say a thing about what she had learned from Ernesto that night sitting on the carpet of their tiny living room, she was deeply and profoundly upset by it.

She dwelled on it constantly. She began running a high fever.

Neither aspirin nor acetaminophen would bring it down. A few weeks later, she started vomiting. No one knew what was wrong. Everyone in the family had always been so healthy.

Then, 3 months after Ernesto's revelations, Sandra started getting black spots on her skin. Ernesto was deeply concerned for her. He called their lawyer, Garcia, who said Ernesto should take Sandra to Louise Ortiz, MD. The doctor's office was in a nice building in the Cherry Creek neighborhood. She examined Sandra and ran blood tests. Three days later she called to report that Sandra's kidneys weren't functioning.

That was mid-2000. The family's asylum was practically assured. Ernesto was married and working a steady job. Things were going well. Why, he asked, when she had been so healthy all of her life, was Sandra suddenly ill? Dr. Ortiz admitted that she had no answers. But Ernesto, looking back, knows. And he knows Sandra knows.

"For so many years," he says in a whisper, his voice trailing off.

Sandra started dialysis. She didn't have any other choice. She had to stay alive. Having been "made legal," she qualified for Medicare and Medicaid, so it wasn't the medical bills that were daunting. It was going three times a week to the dialysis center at Wadsworth and Mississippi to lie there for hours with needles in her veins while machines did for her what her kidneys could not.

Sandra also went through the tests that would put her on the kidney waiting list. The tests confirmed that her kidneys had died. None of the doctors could explain why. No medical reason was ever found.

Organ transplants involve three kinds of legal issues. First, there is the integrity of the human body. Second, there is the authority of the state. And third, there is the ability of the state to project its laws onto actions that take place outside its borders.

When it comes to the integrity of the body, writes Austen Garwood-Gowers in *Living Donor Organ Transplantation: Key Legal and Ethical Issues*, "Medical law in general supports the right to self-determination. Competent adults are given protection from the violation of their body through the general legal right to refuse treatment and take action for criminal assault and/or tortious battery where the medical professional makes an intervention without first obtaining consent, unless this was justified in the deference of rights of others or in an emergency."[1] This premise is honored throughout the United States and those other countries that inherited the "common law" from England.

Most legal studies of organ transplants therefore start with "informed consent," which in the case of transplantation must be obtained from both the recipient and the donor, if alive, or the donor's legal representatives if the donor is cadaveric and has not left definitive instructions about the disposition of his or her body. Topics include the disclosure necessary to satisfy the demands of informed choice, motivation and voluntariness in making an informed choice, the rights of minors and incompetents versus the rights of competent adults, and commerce and compensation.[2]

In addition, cases grounded in constitutional law support the freedoms Americans enjoy when dealing with their own bodies. A competent adult Christian Scientist cannot be forced to accept a blood transfusion under the First Amendment's free exercise clause.[3] American Indians are often exempted from drug laws when ingesting ritual peyote.[4]

In 1965, the Supreme Court struck down laws preventing the use of contraception.[5] This was the beginning of the modern right of privacy. The Court said: "[S]pecific guarantees in the Bill of Rights have penumbras . . . that help give them life and substance. [They] create zones of privacy. The right of association contained in the penumbra of the First Amendment is one. . . . The Fourth Amendment explicitly affirms the 'right of the people to be secure in their persons, houses, papers, and effects, against unreasonable searches and seizures.' The Fifth Amendment . . . enables the citizen to create a zone of privacy which government may not force him to surrender to his detriment."

Eight years later, in *Roe v. Wade*, the Court held: "This right of privacy . . . is broad enough to encompass a woman's decision whether or not to terminate her pregnancy."[6]

The transformation of the right of privacy into a right of bodily self-determination has continued for decades. In 2003 the Supreme Court, now dominated by conservatives, struck down a state's antisodomy law directed at homosexuals.[7] The Court explained: "Liberty protects the person from unwarranted government intrusions into a dwelling or other private places. And there are other spheres of our lives and existence, outside the home, where the State should not be a dominant presence. Freedom extends beyond spatial bounds. Liberty presumes an autonomy of self that includes freedom of thought, belief, expression, and certain intimate conduct."[8]

It's easy to see the connection between this right of privacy and the debates over bodily integrity that arise in the context of organ transplants, and especially in the context of buying and selling organs. Still, there are few rights that are absolute even if they are grounded in the Constitution. The right to bear arms doesn't include the right to own an atomic bomb. Human sacrifice for religious purposes just won't cut it in America.

That means the right of bodily integrity depends on the authority of the state. Ever since the modern "welfare state" was ushered into our lives by the New Deal, Americans have struggled with these competing realities: Constitutionally, we demand a government that is limited in its reach, but socially, economically, and politically, we also expect the government to get more and more involved in our everyday lives.

This tension permeates all of constitutional law. And, just as the integrity of the body cannot be considered without taking into account the authority of the state, so too must we take into account the ability of the state to project its laws onto actions—like the purchase and sale of human organs—that take place outside its borders.

American courts increasingly allow the projection of American laws onto others. Prosecutions for conduct outside US borders involving the smuggling of drugs, arms, and people have become commonplace. Laws against financial crimes that cross the borders of nations are routinely enforced against smugglers and terrorists alike.

Could the United States make it a crime within the reach of its courts for an American citizen to go abroad to buy an organ from a foreigner? This question shows the obvious connection between the legal issues and the political roadblock of sovereignty.

Just what is this thing we call "sovereignty"? Here is one definition:[9]

Sovereignty is the form of political organization that has dominated the international system since the Treaty of Westphalia in 1648. Sovereign states have exclusive and final jurisdiction over territory, as well as the resources and populations that lie within such territory. A system based on sovereignty is one that acknowledges only one political authority over a particular territory and looks to that authority as the final arbiter to solve problems that occur within its border.

Sovereign states have four characteristics, three of which are negotiable: territory, population, a government with control over the territory and population, and international recognition. [O]nly international recognition is non-negotiable. If a political entity has territory, population and a government but lacks international recognition, then it is not . . . a sovereign state.

Six generations after the Treaty of Westphalia, 13 American colonies changed the concept of sovereignty forever. What was truly revolutionary about the American Revolution was the idea of popular sovereignty. "The most novel and crucial American innovation in political thought was the idea of sovereignty of the people."[10]

Finally, during the 20th century, organizations composed of nation-states took on powers and functions formerly reserved for "sovereign" states. The imposition of economic sanctions by trans-sovereign organizations like the United Nations grew to new heights. Justice went international. The war crimes trials at Nuremberg following World War II set enduring precedents.

Over time, the relative nature of sovereignty became accepted. The numbers of quasi-states, failed states, "statelets," pseudo-nations, and conquered nations proliferated. The legal issues blended into the political and economic issues.

And when it comes to economics, globalization still reigns supreme.

Thomas L. Friedman, winner of three Pulitzer Prizes, defines globalization as the "integration of markets, transportation systems, and communications systems to a degree never witnessed before, enabling corporations, countries, and individuals to reach around the world farther, faster, deeper, and cheaper than ever before, and enabling the world to reach into corporations, countries, and individuals farther, faster, deeper, and cheaper. [It] means the spread of free-market capitalism to virtually every country in the world."[11]

The growth of global markets for organs has a deep connection to the processes of globalization. The "commodification" of the body combines with self-determination and the barriers that inhibit intervention in the affairs of others to create the conditions suitable for these organ markets. Economics, politics, and laws rule our lives.

CHAPTER FOUR

THE GOOD LIFE,
THREATENED

I get invited to a lot of events. Sometimes it seems as if I spend more time attending galas, fund-raisers, and photo ops for charities and political candidates than actually practicing law, though the line between the two is hardly fixed.

On a spring night in 2003, I went to an event for the National Kidney Foundation at the home of Bill and Deb MacMillan of the Cargill MacMillan family. Their great wealth came from the family's huge agricultural conglomerate. Deb's father had been among the first recipients of a kidney transplant.

I thought it would be just another night of schmoozing. The event was outdoors. I made the rounds with Cindy. There must have been 300 people standing around the pool, pool house, and tents, listening to the music, eating, drinking, and talking.

Then the music stopped. The fund-raising pitch began. They introduced five kidney transplant donors and recipients. I said to myself, "Boy, they look so normal."

Then I realized I was there for a reason. I felt that strong sense of purpose my mother had infused in me. There was something in the air that night, like a buzz.

I began reflecting, remembering my own kidney disease as an infant.

It was all so vivid: the trip with my parents to the tall, gray buildings at the Mayo Clinic in Rochester, then my abandonment to the nurses at Children's Hospital in Denver, then the "measles cure" and all the rest. But it was all internalized. Cindy was standing right there with me, at my side, also listening to the pitch, but I didn't say anything to her about it. It all went on inside my head. I felt there had to be a connection between this fund-raising event and my own experiences.

I was ripe for the picking when the head of the National Kidney Foundation approached me after the program and suggested I get involved with his organization. Still, I refrained from making a commitment. And because he knew I had worked for many charitable causes in Denver, he did not pressure me.

The things I had thought about that night—the memories that had flooded through me—struck a chord, it was true. But I wanted to reflect on them.

As it turned out, I was swept up in other concerns over the next 3 months. I was representing the developers of a new convention center hotel in Denver, and that demanded a lot of attention. I was the managing partner of our law firm, which had reached more than 100 members and was still growing by leaps and bounds. And to top it off, I was doing fund-raising on behalf of Democratic presidential candidate Senator Joe Lieberman, including holding a dinner party at our home for more than 100 guests.

A lot was going on, but that was typical of my schedule. I wasn't feeling particularly overtaxed or overworked mentally, but I did notice that my level of physical energy seemed diminished. I was feeling sluggish and I didn't recover as quickly after working out or playing tennis. I also noticed that my appetite was down. Still, I thought it was all just part of being too busy and about to turn 60 in a few months. I had never turned 60 before. I figured my metabolism was just slowing down.

In June I went to my doctor, Rick Abrams, MD, for my routine physical. We did heart and lung imaging and they looked fine. Then we did kidney imaging and it showed a lot of scar tissue and cysts, which was not that unusual, given my history. Still, Rick decided to order some blood tests to measure my creatinine level. Creatinine is a by-product of creatine phosphate, a high-energy phosphate-storage compound found in muscles. It is usually filtered by the kidneys. If the kidneys do not filter it properly, its level rises in the blood. The tests Rick ordered came back with bad news. My creatinine level was more than 7. Normal is between 0.8 and 1.5. This was an alarming result. To say that my kidneys were not functioning well would have been an understatement.

Abrams sent me to see Mel Klein, MD, a leading Denver nephrologist whom I knew from having been involved with Denver's Rose Medical Center for years. I had once served as chairman of its board of trustees and I did a lot of fund-raising on its behalf. Getting top medical care was not going to be the problem.

The problem was my kidneys. Dr. Klein ran more tests and soon confirmed how poorly they were functioning. He sent me home on a Friday afternoon with a large, white plastic bottle that I was instructed to urinate into over the course of an entire day. Every drop of my urine output was supposed to go into that bottle. I cheated once, when I went golfing. I refused to carry that bottle with me, so I peed on a tree and it never got put in the bottle. I never knew if it made any difference.

On Monday, I turned in my bottle and soon learned what we already knew: I was suffering from kidney failure. They were functioning at less than 20 percent of normal. That was the reason I had been feeling so tired and sluggish and the reason I had been losing my appetite. My kidneys were starting to shut down.

And to make matters even worse, I was told there was nothing they could do to stop or reverse the process. Two weeks later, I traveled back east to the Johns Hopkins Hospital in Baltimore for more tests and a second opinion, and they agreed with my doctors in Denver.

Operating at a level of less than 20 percent of normal and falling, my kidneys were rapidly deteriorating.

"How rapidly?" I asked.

"Too soon to tell," they said.

"What are my options?" I asked.

"Dialysis or transplant," they said.

"How soon must I decide?" I asked.

"When your functioning falls to 15 percent," they said, "you're dead."

"How soon?" I repeated the question, insistent. I wanted to know exactly what I was facing. I wanted the facts. I got ambiguities.

"Any time between tomorrow and 3 years," they answered.

And there was the rub. Even if I could get on the kidney waiting list immediately, the average waiting time in Colorado was more than 3½ years. I was miserable.

I simply could not bear the thought of going on dialysis. It just was not me; I wouldn't be able to lie still for several hours a day, 3 days a week. It would kill me quicker than the kidney failure.

Jim and Lynne Sullivan traveled with Cindy and me to Johns Hopkins to gather more opinions. Jim is Irish and Catholic, but likes to think of himself as Jewish. He's a fairly big guy, too, like me and my partner, Norm. We all take up a lot of space. We all have a certain presence.

A football player in high school in Chicago, Jim enlisted in the army and saw serious combat in Vietnam. After seeing so much death, he embraces life with exuberance. And he faces his challenges with a certain nonchalance. He has built and lost and rebuilt a major real estate development business and several restaurants.

I met Jim in 1978. Back then, he was a small-time shopping center developer working on a deal with Herb Cook, Cindy's father and the owner of a major chain of sporting goods stores in Denver. Herb liked Jim's energy and invited him to have lunch with us. For years I had been acting as the principal lawyer for Herb's sporting goods chain.

We ate at old Lafittes, with its long, heavy red draperies. At the end of the meal, Herb pulled out cigars and the three of us lit up. Jim noted that I didn't smoke much of mine, but still the two of us hit it off quickly over those cigars. Both of us had grown up without privilege and both of us were working hard to make something of ourselves.

"Steve was successful by then," says Jim now, "but not yet the power broker."

Over the next 10 years we found ourselves doing a lot of "guy things" together. We were both friends with Sidney Schlenker, the owner of the Denver Nuggets basketball team. The Nuggets, like many of the clients of my firm, put me in contact with lots of politicians and celebrities. They were perfect for schmoozing opportunities.

It was during those years—the 1980s—that Jim learned I had been ill as a child. Though I tried not to be self-centered or complain, the story came out in bits and pieces. I had suffered a "hepatitis-like" illness when I was a toddler. That's why I watched what I ate, exercised, and stayed fit. I avoided alcohol and when I did light a cigar, as I had when Jim and I had first met, I would take only a couple of puffs. By the end of the decade, we were close. "Steve was there for me in 1990," says Jim, "when my bankruptcy first got started."

Jim credits me with giving him the best advice he's ever received from any lawyer. When Jim was being deposed in connection with the bankruptcy of his company, he was angry and frustrated. At the end of a tough day, I called him and we met on the street. I could tell he was distressed. "What's wrong?" I asked.

"They want to cut me up and scatter the pieces," said Jim despondently.

"No," I said very gently. "They just want you to settle with them. They want some money now and a promise that you will pay them off over time. That's all."

"That's all?" he asked, a glimmer of hope in his eyes.

"That's all," I repeated.

He sighed. For Jim, it was like getting permission to start on his next life.

Now, as I faced my own crisis, Jim and his wife, Lynne, were there to help me. On this trip to Johns Hopkins, Lynne served as a buffer between me and Cindy, who was so distraught by my predicament that she couldn't hear what was going on. "And I would be there to protect him," says Jim of his role.

It was not until those doctors at Johns Hopkins confirmed my worst fears that the idea of my "life expectancy" became a reality for me. After their exam and consultation, I was feeling pretty introverted. Jim recalls the scene in the waiting room: "There was a sense of definiteness. Lynne was taking notes, Cindy was hysterical, Steve was withdrawn as they all processed what the doctors had just said. Before, they had all denied the severity of the situation to some degree, but now there was no avoiding it."

I needed a kidney transplant. And soon. For me, there was no other choice.

Why should people with kidney failure have to wait so long for a transplant? It's simply because not enough people donate their organs. And while there may be a dramatic shortage of transplant organs, there is no shortage of books, articles, and Web sites about the issue, reflecting a dazzling array of opinions with statistics to back them up.

Among the most reliable of the Web sites for data is the official United Network for Organ Sharing (UNOS) site, www.unos.org. That should certainly be expected. Since 1986 UNOS has held the exclusive contract with the US Department of Health and Human Services to operate America's only Organ Procurement and Transplantation Network (OPTN) under the National Organ Transplant Act (NOTA).

Like the Uniform Anatomical Gift Act (UAGA), which has now been adopted by all the states, NOTA explicitly prohibits the buying and selling of human organs for transplant purposes. The statute makes it a federal crime, punishable with a fine of up to $50,000 and imprisonment for up to 5 years, to acquire, receive, or transfer a human organ for "valuable consideration." Recently an exception was enacted for "human organ paired donation" under the Charlie W. Norwood Living Donation Act. This new exception will be discussed in Chapters Eleven and Twelve, but in short it works like this: Fred wants to give his kidney to his wife, Martha, but is incompatible, while Ethan wants to give his kidney to his wife, Nancy, but is incompatible; Fred is compatible with Nancy, however, and Ethan is compatible with Martha. The new law allows Fred to donate to Nancy in exchange for Ethan donating to Martha.[1]

NOTA applies nationwide, but its implementation is left to the network of regional procurement agencies that make up the OPTN. That means different states and regions have room to experiment. In Pennsylvania, a state-run trust fund now offers the families of deceased organ donors limited payments of funeral expenses. And other states are experimenting with presumed consent laws that allow people to "opt out" of being a donor rather than requiring them to "opt in" if they wish to be.[2] Should we encourage local experiments like these, or do we need a national response? Some people condemn the search for organs. Some even question whether a shortage exists. Nancy Scheper-Hughes, PhD, of the University of California at Berkeley, founded Organs Watch to study the related social, economic, and human rights issues.[3] She has written: "A medically invented, artificial scarcity in human organs for transplantation has generated a kind of panic and a desperate international search for them and for new surgical possibilities."[4]

In 2001, Dr. Scheper-Hughes presented a report to the House Subcommittee on International Operations and Human Rights. The report stated: "The 'demand' for human organs, tissues, and body parts—and the search for wealthy transplant patients to purchase them—is driven by the medical discourse on scarcity. But the very idea of organ 'scarcity' is an artificially created need, invented by transplant technicians and dangled before the eyes of an ever-expanding sick, aging, and dying population."[5]

Dr. Scheper-Hughes is often quoted in the battle against the commercialization of organs. Her verifications and documentations of organ sales and theft are invaluable. But objective she is not. "The ultimate fetish," she has written, "is the idea of 'life' itself as an object of manipulation. This fetishization of life—to be preserved, prolonged and enhanced at almost any cost—erases any possibility of a social ethic. . . . Desperation on both sides and a willingness of the transplant doctors and their patients to see only one side of the transplant equation allows the commodified kidney to become an almost fetishized organ of opportunity for the buyer and an organ of last resort for the seller."[6]

To understand what Dr. Scheper-Hughes means when she says organs have become "commodified" and "fetishized," we turn to Marx. *Das Kapital* describes "the fetishism of commodities and the secret thereof."[7] It says people in capitalist societies "fetishize" material objects. They believe products contain magical powers that consumption imparts to them. Brands of clothing, foods, and perfumes can thus be "fetishized."

In other words, when Dr. Scheper-Hughes questions the scarcity of transplant organs, her views are loaded with assumptions. And another word for those assumptions is "bias." In her case, it would be too easy to write off her assumptions—her bias—as the natural consequence of being a radical leftist anthropologist from Berkeley. However, her bias was formed after decades of deep research into and writing about the effects of violence on the poor, and her opinions are well respected. Besides, everything written about this subject is biased. Everyone has an agenda. But sound public policy requires multidisciplinary decision making in a political environment.

That means everyone with a bias and an agenda should be heard. All the statistics, data, and opinions should be gathered. The religious, moral, and ethical concerns should all be addressed. And the economic, political, and legal issues should be fully aired.

Then, real, practical decisions should be made without further delay. Over 99,000 Americans are waiting for life-saving transplant organs, and more than 6,500 will die while waiting this year. We can no longer ignore these numbers, nor can we make our decisions solely with regard to personal anecdotes or the plights of particular individuals.

Former Colorado governor Richard D. Lamm has written: "What health care would you deny if it were your mother? My answer: Deny her nothing! Of course we all would do everything to save a loved one. But you cannot build a health care system, or any public system, a mother at a time. This is an unfair and unrealistic standard for public policy. That road leads to national bankruptcy. The 'mother test' is a good yardstick for your own money but is not a sustainable yardstick for a health plan."[8]

Public policy must create enforceable standards for individual conduct that go beyond statistics and anecdotes, beyond theories and labels, to address the religious, ethical, economic, political, and legal parts of the crisis. And a crisis it is.

The current allocation system, with its regional networks of organ procurement organizations and complex rules and donor-matching criteria, simply doesn't do enough. In 1999, the Department of Health and Human Services published its final rule on the OPTN.[9] It created the system of cadaveric organ procurement and allocation that still exists today. Ten years of operating under the final rule have resulted in the disappointing statistics cited above.

The problem is not religion.

All major religions accept the desirability of saving life through organ transplants. Some argue over the meaning of "brain death," but all agree that donation is allowed.[10] Baptists, Episcopalians, Lutherans, Presbyterians, and Catholics all openly encourage organ donations. On June 20, 1991, Pope John Paul II told the First International Congress of the Society of Organ Sharing, "The Catholic church would promote the fact that there is a need for organ donors and that Christians should accept this as a challenge to their generosity and fraternal love so long as ethical principles are followed."[11]

So, too, do all major branches of Judaism encourage organ donation. In 1991 the Orthodox Rabbinical Council deemed organ donations allowable and even required, despite Jewish proscriptions against desecration of the body. Rabbi Moses Tendler, who was then the chairman of the biology department at New York City's Yeshiva University, wrote, "If one is in the position to donate an organ to save another's life, it's obligatory to do so."[12]

Similarly, one survey of Islamic law states the emerging consensus: "It is possible to summarize Islamic views on organ transplant by pointing out the underlying principle of saving human life. Donation of organs from both living and dead has been regarded as permissible in the jurisprudence. However, the prerequisite in the case of a living person is that his/her life is not endangered, whereas in the case of a dead person there must exist his last will or testament permitting thus, or the permission of his relatives."[13]

Buddhists believe that organ donation is a "matter of personal conscience and place high value on acts of compassion."[14] And ancient

Hindu mythology "has stories in which the parts of the human body are used for the benefit of other humans and society. There is nothing in the Hindu religion indicating that parts of humans, dead or alive, cannot be used to alleviate the suffering of other humans."[15]

It seems that few religions actually prohibit organ donation. The Shinto believes the dead body to be impure, dangerous, and powerful, so injuring a dead body is a crime. Cadaveric donation is not allowed. Nothing is said, however, about live organ donation.[16]

So Americans' hesitancy to donate organs cannot be blamed on religion. What about ethics? If morality embedded in religion isn't the answer, then what about morality embedded in ethics? *The Ethics of Organ Transplants* offers 35 essays on the subject, from "The Myth of Presumed Consent" to "Kidney Transplantation from Unrelated Living Donors."[17] Eight of the essays are about commodification, and among them the array of opinions is wide. And that is only one of the many books on the subject.[18]

H. T. Engelhardt Jr., PhD, a professor of philosophy at Rice University in Houston, holds doctorates in philosophy and medicine, has written many books and articles on the subject, and identifies his teaching areas as "Kant, Hegel, philosophy of medicine, and bioethics." He writes that there are five kinds of ethical issues: First, there are issues regarding the moral authority of individuals. The more people demand to have authority over themselves, the more necessary it is to gain their permission for the transfer of their organs, and the harder it is to justify the prohibition of peaceable sales. Second, there are issues regarding the moral authority of states. If states maintain moral authority over their subjects, then it appears to be ethical for them to prohibit peaceable sales. Third, there are issues regarding the commodification of organs. If market exchanges are the key to peaceable mutual respect, then the acquisition of organs through sales can seem to be noble. Fourth are issues regarding the nature and moral implications of economic exploitation. If personal autonomy is seen as crucial or the sale of human body parts as evil, then views will differ about who would be exploiting whom. Finally, there are issues regarding the impact of particular policies because the empirical concerns are often speculative and too difficult to assess.[19]

Simply put: The ethical issues easily blur into the legal, economic, and political debates. Once more, we must confront the three great forces that drive today's events.

CHAPTER FIVE

BROTHERLY LOVE

Sandra waited on the organ transplant list. One millennium passed into another. Then, 2001 gave way to 2002. Every time she walked to the dialysis center and waited for the machines to cleanse her blood, she pondered her predicament.

Sandra never liked to think about her life in Guatemala. After Ernesto had gone to America, she had missed him and cried a lot. She had wanted to go to America, too, and was elated when she finally could. Later, when she first heard Ernesto's story about their parents, she had felt troubled. Then, upset. She had seemed normal physically, but soon those black spots had begun to appear all over her legs and arms.

As Sandra began feeling sick—having the shakes and getting weak—she became convinced that her physical decline was connected to Ernesto's story. She refused to talk about it, however. Then, after months of thinking about it during her dialysis treatments, she approached Ernesto. She asked him, "Why did our parents die?"

When he couldn't give her a good answer, she would wait a day or two, then ask him again. It happened over and over. He was never able to answer her question, any more than her doctors could ever say with assurance what had caused her kidneys to fail.

Finally, in 2003, the doctors insisted that Sandra needed a transplant—and soon. She was not moving up on the organ waiting list and she could not stay on dialysis forever. Her condition would begin to deteriorate without a transplant.

Ernesto, ever the older brother, immediately got tested to see if he was a match. Edgar did not. The idea of donating his kidney to Sandra frightened him.

"He was afraid," says Ernesto, shaking his head and flashing his big, white smile.

Wasn't Ernesto afraid? "Well, maybe a little bit," he admits.

But he had plenty of time to think about it. From the time he first got tested—it takes weeks to undergo the series of tests—until the time he donated his kidney to Sandra, 1 year passed, with the family waiting and hoping she would move up on the waiting list and qualify for a cadaveric kidney. A lot happened. There were more forms to complete, just to qualify for the procedure. Ernesto's daughter, Roselea Galilea, named for her grandmother, turned 4. He expanded the landscaping business he had started in 2000 while working for a major Denver real estate developer, who by pure coincidence happened to be my friend Jim Sullivan.

During that year, Sandra stopped struggling with the demons of her past and started struggling with the threats to her present. She was scared. At first she was scared for herself. Later, she became scared for Ernesto. She worried obsessively: If something were to happen to him, then little Galilea would grow up without a father.

But all the while, Ernesto knew deep down inside that there was only one solution. He had to donate his kidney to Sandra. Why bother to save her from the right-wing death squads in Guatemala in 1984 only to let her die in America 20 years later?

For him, there was no hand-wringing. His choice was clear. He knew that dialysis wasn't a permanent solution. It extends your life by killing you slowly, or so he had heard. At the very least it "cuts down on your life," he says, and over time it makes you less able to successfully receive a transplant.

Ernesto's concerns were well founded. Common side effects of dialysis include low blood pressure, fatigue, chest pains, leg cramps, nausea, and headaches. These are often called "dialysis hangover." There is also a greater risk of infection and, over time, various types of heart disease, including congestive heart failure, enlargement of the heart, and other conditions that make it harder for the patient to later accept a donated kidney. In Sandra's case, over the time from when she first went on dialysis until she received Ernesto's kidney, she lost 50 pounds, going from 135 to 85.

"And she was pretty small to begin with," says Ernesto.

Three times a week, in all sorts of weather, Sandra would walk the 6 blocks from the family home to the dialysis clinic at Wadsworth and Mississippi, and three times a week Ernesto would pick her up afterward. Every time she would be tired.

"She'd sleep all day," says Ernesto. "She wouldn't smile. She felt terrible."

Everyone was feeling bad for Sandra. Ernesto's wife offered to donate her own kidney if that would help. "They were very close, like sisters," he explains. "They had always lived together in the same village or the same house. And Gicela would have freely given her kidney to Sandra if I had not."

But Ernesto was a perfect match for his sister. He learned that siblings are almost always the best match—usually better than parents or children—because their genetic makeup is so nearly identical. Recall that the first successful transplants involved identical twins. The battery of tests that were given to Ernesto to confirm that he was a match for Sandra took almost 4 months. "They tested my blood and my pee and my vision," recalls Ernesto, "and the strength, the pressure, of my breath."

Meanwhile, the family kept waiting and hoping Ernesto would not have to give his kidney to her. Asked if he had alternatives—such as going abroad to buy a kidney—he says he couldn't have done it, but he has no problem with it. Peasants don't have the choices power brokers have. He says that if Sandra's kidneys had failed in his native country, she never would have survived. A kidney transplant wouldn't have been possible. So for him it was a miracle: He was able to come to America and get a transplant for his sister!

With little ado, Ernesto completed all the paperwork that was necessary to donate his kidney to his sister. He never complained—he never does: "There really wasn't that much paperwork. Mostly it was just insurance forms and consent forms. They gave us a caseworker to help us. She seemed very young, about 23. She was skinny, with long legs and black hair. She was from Honduras so she could speak Spanish. She spoke Spanish with us most of the time. She led us through the entire process."

Still, it was Sandra who hesitated. "She didn't want to put any of us in danger," Ernesto explains. "She kept saying that we had to wait for someone else—to die and be the donor, she meant."

All that changed in the spring of 2004. It was a Monday morning. Sandra awoke feeling sicker and weaker than usual. She was scheduled to go for dialysis at 11:00 a.m., but she was feeling too sick to wait for that. She had been drinking a lot of liquids but was not urinating, so her body was filling up with fluids and toxins. Her hands and limbs were shaking. She could not stand by herself.

Ernesto was already driving to work when Sandra called him on his cell phone. "Please—take me to the hospital," she said in a trembling voice.

He heard the panic in her voice, immediately turned around, drove back home, and took her to the emergency room at the University of Colorado Hospital. The emergency room doctor was a young "Spanish guy" from Ecuador. He talked to the brother and sister in Spanish, then he called for a kidney doctor.

"They put her on the machine right there," says Ernesto.

By then Sandra was feeling confused and lightheaded.

She kept asking the doctors, "What's going on?"

The doctors told her she needed dialysis immediately. She could not wait even a little while for her scheduled appointment. They told her the longer she was on dialysis, the harder it would be on her. She was finally at the point where a crisis like this could happen again at any time. Her need for a transplant was acute.

The ER episode on that spring morning tipped the balance for the Delarocas. They knew without saying that they had to get the transplant done for Sandra, and soon. Ernesto gathered the family together in their Lakewood home. This time it was in the family room, not the living room, and this time Garcia the lawyer wasn't there, but Sandra, Edgar, Gicela, and Ernesto were joined by their nephew Raul.

Ernesto told Sandra she had to face the facts. She wasn't moving up on the list. "You're dying," he said. "You can't keep waiting. You have to have the transplant."

Sandra nodded sheepishly. She understood the reality. But she still could not bring herself to actually ask Ernesto to take the next step. He took her off the hook.

"I am giving you my kidney," he said firmly, "and that's all there is to it."

So finally, after her trip to the emergency room and with everyone's urging, Sandra agreed that she was ready to have the surgery. She was ready to let Ernesto save her life once again. The meeting was very emotional, he recalls.

"She finally said okay, so the next day I called the nurse we'd been dealing with. Her first name was Anita. I can't remember her last name. She was American, older, probably somewhere in her fifties. A big woman, plump, with gray hair. She told us she also had gotten a transplant some years before, so she also had only one kidney."

Ernesto was ordered to take more tests.

The surgery was scheduled for 3 weeks later.

Meanwhile, the Human Rights Camp waged war against the Free Market Camp. To human rights activists, the idea of buying and selling transplant organs is abominable. And they may have a point. My own search for a healthy kidney came to resemble a "fetishizing" of the organ. The group of intimates that formed around me was like something out of J. R. R. Tolkien's *Fellowship of the Ring*, with that kidney starring as the ring.

There I was, the king in disguise, trying to do what was right, but having to stay alive to do it. Then came Cindy, my wife, well dressed and well distracted, but deep into her own denial, apart from her king. Add Jim and Lynne Sullivan, our close friends, stout and gracious respectively, the tough Vietnam vet and his tough, no-nonsense wife. Next came Jimmy Lustig, my brother-in-law, and Lee Alpert, my longtime friend.

All of us were worldly and successful, but stepping into an adventure we weren't ready for. It reeked of melodrama and privilege. Yet there was nothing unreal about it.

The members of the Human Rights Camp, led by Dr. Nancy Scheper-Hughes of Organs Watch, would certainly find in my example all the evils they abhor. And make no mistake, despite all the inroads made by the Free Market Camp, the perspective held by the Human Rights Camp remains the dominant one in the world today. The vast majority of nations have laws prohibiting the buying and selling of transplant organs. And more and more countries are joining that majority.

The deep moral revulsion connected with the buying and selling of human organs ranks high among other strongly held beliefs: Slavery is wrong. Child prostitution is wrong. Torture is wrong.

Genocide is wrong. Some things are just plain wrong. They need not refer to any other reasons to justify why they are wrong.

But suppose you disagree. Suppose you think the case is not so clear once you consider the lives that are lost. You are willing to listen to arguments that are not so absolutist.

The Human Rights Camp is ready for you. They are ready to go beyond simplistic thinking to engage you intellectually and emotionally based on the evidence they have gathered. They are ready to say that payment of money for organs is wrong *because* it leads to the exploitation of the poor and the disadvantaged, especially in poor countries; it leads to abuses like theft and fraud; it generates additional wrongs.

Dr. Scheper-Hughes is not alone in her opposition to organ trafficking. But she is perhaps the most articulate and the most frequently quoted. She says, "The growth of 'medical tourism' for transplant surgery . . . has exacerbated older divisions between North and South, and between haves and have-nots. In general, the flow of organs, tissues, and body parts follows the modern routes of capital: from South to North, from third to first world, from poor to rich, from black and brown to white, and from female to male bodies."[1]

She describes how several disadvantaged groups—executed prisoners in China, the mentally retarded, poor patients in public hospitals—have been exploited by the organ trade. Her presentations are filled with compelling anecdotes and statistics that focus on race, class, and gender inequalities. Specific cases of kidney theft and entrapment are detailed.

Eventually, however, her biases show through:[2]

The specter of long transplant "waiting lists"—often we have found only virtual lists with little material basis in reality— has motivated and driven questionable practices of organ harvesting with blatant sales alongside "compensated gifting";

doctors acting as brokers; and fierce competition between public and private hospitals for patients of means. . . . Bio-ethical arguments about the right to sell are based on Euro-American notions of contract and individual "choice." But the social and economic contexts make the "choice" to sell a kidney in an urban slum of Calcutta or in a Brazilian favela anything but a "free" and "autonomous" one. . . . A market price on body parts—even a fair one—exploits the desperation of the poor, turning their suffering into an opportunity.

The studies do, in fact, support these arguments. One study, frequently cited, appeared in the *Journal of the American Medical Association* in 2002 and focused on the economic and health consequences of selling a kidney in India. Others have tracked the consequences of selling a kidney in Iran. These studies are discussed in greater detail in Chapter Seven. But, for now, their conclusions are strikingly consistent and clear: Donating an organ is certainly more dangerous in Third World countries. Postoperative complications are far more likely to occur in such places. Those who have documented kidney donors' lives in countries like India and Iran have also found that their standards of living are seldom made better by the meager compensation they were given in exchange for their organs. Often, it's worse. And they find that the emotional lives of those who have sold a kidney also suffer.

Still, Debra Satz, PhD, of Stanford writes:

"[K]idney markets are worrying to the extent that they involve dangerous risks which might place people below a certain threshold, deepen class and status inequalities, and undermine norms of fairness. [But] we need more empirical research into the actual risks of kidney donation, especially in poor countries. While there is much heated assertion about kidney markets on both sides of the argument, and some rather sensationalist reporting of organ markets generally, the systematic sociological study of these sales actually remains to be carried out. Much depends on empirical facts we have insufficient evidence about and much depends on empirical conjectures."[3]

In other words, according to critics like Dr. Satz, the Human Rights Camp has carried the day, so far, by sensationalizing individual anecdotes, conducting research that is neither complete nor definitive, denying transplant organ scarcity—even denying the very existence of waiting lists! There must be another side to the story. And of course there is. The Free Market Camp has counterattacked the Human Rights Camp, seeking to elevate the principles of economics over all other forces.

Nowhere is this more evident than in the digital pages of the *New York Times*, where the popular *Freakonomics* blog extols the common sense of organ markets.[4]

And beyond the multitude of Web sites arguing the virtues of markets for organs, a wide array of doctors, lawyers, and economists argue that compensating organ donors should not be precluded altogether. As early as 1989, Henry B. Hansmann, PhD, of the Yale Law School proclaimed, "It is possible that a relatively modest financial incentive would improve donation rates substantially. . . . [I]t seems plausible that appeals to altruism, community spirit, and financial self-interest could all be combined in a fashion that would be complementary and effective in securing donations."[5]

Economists have joined the fray with models, charts, and graphs to show that a free market in kidneys would be both efficient and equitable. Indeed, kidneys are best for testing the economists' theories— the paradigm organ—because they can be taken from a live donor and are the organ most often transplanted. The big numbers they would generate would make the test results statistically significant.

It is unsurprising that some of the most passionate of the Free Market Camp hail from the University of Chicago. Merging law and economics became the religion and the trademark of that university in the second half of the 20th century. The impact of that merger is seen almost everywhere today.

The law and economics movement shows up in the opinions of US Seventh Circuit Court of Appeals judge Richard Posner. It shows up in the works of Nobel Prize winner Milton Friedman and in the detailed cost-benefit analysis that characterizes America's regulatory approach to problems. It is evident in the way we seek to put values on things like trees and rivers and air so we can then subject them to the rigors of formulas and theories. It has become the dominant mode of thought in law schools throughout the country and the dominant mode of policy analysis in graduate schools of government.[6]

The Human Rights Camp may have held sway thus far when it comes to payments for transplant organs, but the Free Market Camp—led by the Chicago school—has captured the imagination of makers of law and policy everywhere else. The Chicago school attacks the Human Rights Camp directly, often with dueling statistics and competing rhetoric about the greater good.[7]

One of the most vocal advocates for a market approach was David L. Kaserman, PhD, who served at the Federal Trade Commission and the US Department of Housing and Urban Development. (Dr. Kaserman passed away in January 2008 after a kidney transplant.) His 2002 book with economist A. H. Barnett, *The U.S. Organ Procurement System*, is filled with charts, graphs, and statistics of the kind that make the Chicago school break out in smiles. Dr. Kaserman and Barnett argue that the shortage of organs has persisted for decades and something must be done about it. They believe that the findings demonstrate the desirability, on social welfare grounds, of repealing the NOTA ban on cadaveric organ sales.

"That ban," they said, "has caused the unnecessary deaths of tens of thousands of patients and prolonged the suffering of thousands more." They add that our current cadaveric organ procurement policy kills patients while increasing costs. And all of this is done for "the high moral purpose" of preventing the families of recently deceased accident victims from receiving any payment for agreeing to allow the removal of their loved ones' organs. The authors conclude with this dark thought: "It is, frankly, difficult to imagine a crueler, more perverse system of procurement."[8]

Dr. Kaserman and Barnett acknowledge that some Indians who sold their kidneys reported having had bad health experiences afterward, and so did some Iranians. Many said that if they could do it over, they would not sell their organs. The authors say, however, that the experience in these two poor nations is not comparable to what would happen in the United States or other advanced nations. They argue that the quality of the surgery would be far superior, as would both pre- and postoperative care, though in this day of "transplant tourism," these assertions seem conclusory. It is true, nevertheless, that the experience in the United States indicates that the subsequent health of kidney donors is very good, and there is little reason to expect a worse experience for those who get paid.

Armed with their statistics, assumptions, arguments—and bias—the two economists propose their own version of a free market system. Here's how their system would work: Organ suppliers—potential donors or their surviving family members—would be offered a market-determined price (which would fluctuate with changes in supply and demand) by procurement firms in exchange for permission to remove transplantable organs at death. Those firms would then sell the harvested organs to transplant centers that have placed orders with them. The center would include the price paid in the bill for the transplant operation, just as all other inputs are billed. In a truly competitive environment, the resale price would equal the price paid to the donor or family plus the marginal cost to the firm of collecting and distributing the organ. This additional cost could be covered by Medicare for kidney transplants or by insurance companies for other organs. Once the organs are purchased, the transplant center would allocate them to recipients in the same way that they are allocated today under the United Network for Organ Sharing rules.[9]

This market-based solution is limited to cadaveric organs because Dr. Kaserman and Barnett believe that modest payments to cadaveric organ sellers would be sufficient to lift the supply to meet the demand. Today, many in the Free Market Camp go even further and argue in favor of creating markets for live organs and payments to living organ providers. For there is little doubt, when it comes to kidneys, that fresher is better. And the freshest are live.

It all sounds so ghoulish: "harvesting" and "marginal cost."

No wonder there are reformers seeking to find a workable solution somewhere between the extremes of the Human Rights Camp and the Free Market Camp.

PART TWO

A SYSTEM IN DISTRESS

CHAPTER SIX

THE AMERICAN TRANSPLANT SYSTEM

I needed that new kidney. Within a couple of weeks of my diagnosis, my doctor, Mel Klein, referred me to the transplant center at the University of Colorado Health Sciences Center. I talked to several doctors on their staff. Soon, I made my way to Larry Chan, MD, the head of renal transplant medicine. During the process, I was assigned a caseworker named Tara Morgan. She was young, maybe 26, and had recently had a baby. She was also the first person who put together multiple pieces of the puzzle for me. She was just terrific.

Tara told me what I had to do to get on the waiting list. She was very frank. She said my position on that list would have nothing to do with whatever money, power, or influence I had. The determining factors would be the availability of a matching organ and my time on the waiting list. Unlike the case of liver transplants, my deteriorating medical condition would not be a factor.

I learned just how precious human transplant organs are. They are not "wasted" on people who aren't good candidates for transplantation. Good candidates, to the transplant community, are generally people who will likely recover and lead healthy and productive lives after their transplants. If, for example, you have cancer or some sort of metabolic disorder or immune system syndrome that will likely interfere with your ability to fully "use" a transplanted organ, they probably won't even put you on the list. To its credit, however, the medical community is always trying to expand the pool of good candidates with research and improved techniques.

So I had to be examined and tested thoroughly. It took a lot of time—more than 2 months—before I even got on the list, and time was not my friend.

I was getting sicker and sicker. I was feeling worse and worse. It wasn't a matter of pain, but rather something that seemed worse to me—weakness, sluggishness, fatigue. I was dwelling on my declining condition. I was getting around, but it was getting harder and harder.

The biopsies were the worst. They biopsied each of my organs, everything from my liver to my skin. The biopsy for prostate cancer was the worst of the worst. Picture a 1½-liter bottle of water—something that big around—shoved up your rectum with no sedation and only some local anesthesia. Then they go in and take chunks of whatever they want—*snip! snip!*—and you feel it and you hear it and it's very painful, and by the time it is over you are soaked in blood.

Meanwhile, with all my shuffling back and forth from one hospital to the next and all the tests, procedures, and consultations, rumors were flying throughout the Denver Jewish, social, and legal communities. I must be very sick, they surmised. Some said I could be dying. Now, this was not particularly surprising since I am a fairly high-profile person.

Then there was my law firm. People told people, and the next thing I knew, rumors were flying there, too. We were having growing pains. We were healthy in terms of our business, clients, and culture, but the question of leadership in the next generation was presenting itself. Norm Brownstein had turned 60 already and I was turning 60 in September. The question of phasing us out and phasing in new leadership had come up over the years, but had never been pressed. After all, Norm and I continued to bring in the lion's share of the firm's business.

This time, however, was different. The growing pains were challenging our tempers and our moods. One day that summer, two of my partners came to me and said, "We heard you are dying." It was that direct.

"I am not dying," I said to them, "but I do need a kidney transplant."

"Well, everyone knows something is going on," they replied, "so maybe we should send an e-mail or something to the lawyers."

I looked at them with disbelief. They wanted to send the lawyers an e-mail?

That was not the right thing to do.

So I called all the lawyers in the Denver office together and the first thing I said to them was this: "My points are not available and neither is my office."

It was just a joke. In our firm, partner compensation is based on how many "points" you have—which in turn is based on seniority, productivity, acquisition of new clients, and other factors—and if a partner leaves, there's a feeding frenzy over his or her points. It's not like a bunch of sharks. It's more like a school of piranhas.

The joke worked. It broke the ice. Everyone laughed.

Then I told them all about my kidney condition, as honestly as I could. I asked them for their support and they gave it, one and all. It was really very touching.

Next, I gathered together all the staff—at the time there were more than 100 of them—and told them about my condition as well. They had heard the rumors, of course. And I never saw 100 more appreciative faces than the faces of those people that day. They were glad it was all out in the open, that they had been included, that it was now okay for them to give me their support, too.

That summer was really something. I was getting tested to get on the waiting list. There was turmoil at the firm. My condition was declining. It was all so exhausting.

Finally, in August, I got on the list. I felt relieved. A big hurdle had been cleared. But now I faced a new challenge: waiting on the list. And I'm not good at waiting.

In September, Cindy and I traveled to Italy with Jim and Lynne Sullivan to celebrate my 60th birthday. Sitting on the gracious veranda at the Palazzo Sasso in Ravello, with the late afternoon sun sparkling off the emerald Gulf of Salerno and the red-roofed buildings casting their shadows on the towns below, I thought about my situation.

I was feeling pretty weak physically and not much better emotionally. I started contemplating my death. I realized it was possible that it could arrive a lot sooner than I had ever expected. I feared this birthday trip might be my last hurrah.

Jim had not wanted to go on the trip because he had an infection in his leg, but he knew he had to. It wasn't that I insisted on it, or because we had even really talked about it, but because he knew that I was afraid this birthday would be my last. Toward the end of the trip, the mood turned serious. We were all going back to face an unpleasant reality. On my birthday, Jim recalls, "We were sitting outside at this little café in Ravello. It was the feast of Santa Maria. Below us stretched the rugged Amalfi Coast. We were at the top of the cliff, overlooking the scene. Fireworks were going off and they were spectacular. Steve took significance in how scenic and beautiful it was. He said, 'I may never get to see this again.' He was resolved to his fate."

Lynne Sullivan, Jim's wife, has always been a very spiritual woman. She is deeply interested in alternative healing and medicine. Still, she is neither a New Age airhead nor a typical trophy wife. She is very well read, well versed, and well traveled. Proudly brunette in a sea of bottled blondes, she is statuesque and commanding. The survivor of a spectacular head-on collision with a drunk driver, she is strong, thoughtful, and grounded. Lynne more than matches Jim, and he's a character.

Lynne was always the one who kept Jim—and all the rest of us—channeled. I could get lost in my personal dramas and medical dilemmas, in my struggle for life itself. Lynne was the rock, the one who listened carefully to the doctors' explanations and took copious notes. Cindy could go hysterical all she wanted, because Lynne would bring her back down to Planet Earth.

Lynne chuckles as she confirms, "Yes, it's true. We were the best friends of the king and queen of the Jews in Denver."

During the months before and after my surgery, she talked to me every day. I was very private and didn't want the whole city to know all of my medical problems. But with Lynne, I found that I could really open up. "Cindy and Jim are a lot alike," explains Lynne. "They shop, they emote, they live for the moment. They're playful."

Playful? Does she really think that my wife, Cindy, is playful?

"Yes," Lynne insists. "Much of what people see of her is all just public persona—wife, mother, daughter, social magnate. But privately, she can be fun.

"By contrast," says Lynne, "Steven and I are more alike."

She almost always calls me Steven, not Steve. It seems to fit our relationship. We are both very levelheaded, linear, and more down to earth than our spouses. When we used to travel together—and we used to travel together quite frequently—Lynne and I would get up hours before Cindy and Jim so we could have breakfast together, then take a long walk and plan the day.

"You know when you toss a pebble into water?" Lynne asks. "How it makes ripples in circles and the circles get bigger and bigger the farther they go from where the pebble was dropped? Well, the Farbers' social life is like that. There are very, very few people who get inside that innermost circle. A lot of the women Cindy grew up with in Denver call her all the time, just to check in, just to be part of the circle, even if it is a bigger and less intimate circle. And a lot of people all over Denver want to ride on the coattails of Steven and Cindy Farber."

When Lynne first met Cindy, the brunette shiksa who had been living in the mountains didn't know what to make of the blonde queen-in-training. Lynne assumed she and Cindy would not have much in common. Over time, Lynne was proved wrong.

"I learned over time," says Lynne, "that Cindy has a temperament and personality that are very different from her persona."

Cindy and Lynne saw each other often at social events. They got to know each other better, even as Jim and I were forming our own separate friendship. The two women realized they actually had a lot in common. Both had grown up wealthy. Both had married men who had come from nowhere—men who had built their own positions out of nothing. Both had three sons and similar values when it came to mothering.

The turning point in Lynne and Cindy's relationship came during the weekend when Sidney Schlenker, the owner of the Denver Nuggets, flew Jim, Lynne, Cindy, and me to Houston for the NBA All-Stars Game. It was pure first-class, VIP treatment.

On the ride from the airport to the sports arena—I remember that Lynne called it the "dome-thingy"—our little bus passed through the swanky Galleria shopping area. Now, this was before the Cherry Creek Shopping Center brought swanky shopping to Denver.

"Well," says Lynne, "Cindy and I saw all those shops we didn't have back home. We took one look at each other and that's all there was to it. We said, 'Stop the bus. Right here. Right now. We're getting out.' Jim and Steven looked at us like we were both from outer space. 'We're almost there and you want to stop?' they both asked, shaking their heads. And sure enough, we did."

After that trip to Houston, Lynne and Cindy started talking on the phone and seeing more of each other. They attended social gatherings together. Lynne began to connect as much with me as with Cindy.

"Steven and I think a lot alike," says Lynne. "I can understand him. Oftentimes, I lose the train of thought when I talk to Cindy or Jim."

On the evening before I went to have body imaging done as part of my yearly physical—the event that triggered my awareness that I was having kidney problems—I mentioned to Lynne that I was having it done. The next day she asked, "How'd it go?"

I answered, "I just don't know, Lynny. It showed that one of my kidneys isn't working too well."

Lynne immediately clicked into action. She started to research the various types of renal failure on the Internet. She searched for specific answers to specific questions: At what point do you have to go on dialysis? At what point do you need a transplant?

"As visible as he is," says Lynne, "Steven is a very private person. He wanted to keep his condition as quiet as he possibly could. So he and I talked about it privately. We talked about what I was learning from my research. I went through all of it with him, from start to finish. Like he says, the test they gave him for prostate cancer was by far the worst. He came out afterward covered in blood."

Lynne would take notes at doctors' appointments because she is close, but not a member of the immediate family; she is good at being a facilitator; she is good at gathering information; and she is good at asking questions. I was much too close to the problem; it was my body that was rebelling, after all. And neither Jim nor Cindy had the temperament.

So Lynne accepted her role as my medical advocate without hesitation.

After our fateful visit to Johns Hopkins, when our worst fears were confirmed, Lynne tried to talk to Cindy about some of the specifics: what we all could expect over the next year, dialysis, transplants—all the details. But Cindy just couldn't think beyond the reality that, without a new kidney, I would die. And later, the protective mother in her couldn't face the reality that her son might have to donate one of his kidneys so I could live.

Lynne completely understood Cindy's motherly impulse to avoid at all costs having her son as the donor. She learned to tread lightly. When my 60th birthday was approaching, she asked me what I wanted to do to celebrate it. I told her that I didn't want a big party. I wanted to keep it private. So the four of us had gone to Italy and then came home to face those realities she had tried to discuss with Cindy.

Now my daily visits with Lynne increased in their intensity. It was October and I still had not moved up on the waiting list. Without my knowledge or consent, people in the community—powerful people who supported charitable causes with big donations—called on Jim Shore, MD, who was then the head of the University of Colorado Health Sciences Center, to better understand the system and, perhaps, get me moved up on the list. I met with him twice myself to learn more about the system.

Cindy, Jim, and my partner, Norm Brownstein, went to see Dr. Shore to find out if anything could be done. Jim says, "We went to beg for Steve's life. Cindy was very emotional and far too combative. Norm was proper, exact, and forceful. He was trying to empower Jim Shore intellectually—trying to help him find a reason why he could move Steve up on the waiting list. I was there, once again, as the enforcer. We tried to impress upon Jim Shore everything he already knew: Steve was not only very important to his family and friends, but to his community and the hospital itself. Steve and Norm were the ones who often went to Washington and pitched for dollars for the university."

Dr. Shore told them he would get back to them after he looked over my case. When he did, the message was clear: The only factors that would move me up on the list would be the availability of a matching organ and my time waiting on the list; even my deteriorating medical condition would not count. He explained: The big controversy over the liver transplant given to baseball legend Mickey Mantle—who was recovering from longtime alcoholism and had other conditions that made him less suitable than others for a transplant—had made the transplant committee extremely sensitive to any charges of submitting to influence, money, or power in moving someone up on the waiting list. That option was absolutely unavailable. No special dispensation could be given. Favoritism was out of the question. *There would be no more Mickey Mantles!*

So I could wait for 3½ years—the average wait in Colorado at the time—hoping in the meantime that I wouldn't die or have to go on dialysis to stay alive. Or, I could move to a state like Florida, where the average wait for a kidney transplant at that time was only 12 months. By then I had learned that different states have different waiting times depending on their rates of death, donation, and demand—as well as myriad other factors. Suffice it to say, demand is greatest in cities with concentrated populations. Geography doesn't favor them. But for me to take advantage of the shorter wait in Florida, I would have to actually move there, and my firm, my clients, and my family could not tolerate that.

I had one other choice: I could find my own live donor, someone who could be approved as a "match." That's because the waiting list applies only to cadaveric organs.

That meant there was no wait with a live donor! So the call went out. And the response was overwhelming. More than 50 people offered to get tested to see if they could be a donor for me. And they were not just my relatives. Former Colorado senator Hank Brown— my pledge father in my college fraternity—was turned away for being too old. Unfortunately, a lot of my peers were older than me, and to maximize the transplant's odds of success, I needed a younger donor. So, many people who offered simply didn't qualify. In other cases, people who offered to get tested never did. One told me he wanted to, but his daughter forbade him from risking his life for me. Still others came out of the woodwork, offering herbal remedies, water purifiers, diets, recipes, and even faith healers. I went on the Johns Hopkins diet, which is very low in protein, though when I talked to the doctor who created it, he insisted it would not solve my problem. I might feel better on it, but I would still need a new kidney.

Of all the people who were tested, my 32-year-old son, Gregg, was the best possible donor. His tests showed he was a six-antigen match: perfect compatibility. But I was very reluctant to put his health at risk, and Cindy, always the fiercely protective mother, was adamantly opposed to it. I had to find a kidney somewhere else.

By late autumn, I was feeling overwhelmed and frustrated. I was not moving up on the waiting list and Cindy was still opposing Gregg's donation. I had entered a labyrinth of medical, legal, and ethical problems. My route was tortured and circuitous. It had none of the humble elegance of Ernesto's journey through the maze. I was wringing my hands over what to do while learning more about the system.

As a lawyer I could understand the interplay between the Uniform Anatomical Gift Act (UAGA) and the National Organ Transplant Act (NOTA) on an intellectual level. But the confusing relationship between state and federal statutes as well as all the specific guidelines and criteria and regulations governing organ allocation—they were hard to take on an emotional level. And, I thought, if it was hard for me, imagine what it must be like for people who were not used to reading statutes and cases.

What's worse, the Organ Procurement and Transplant Network operates on a regional basis. There are 11 regions. Colorado is in Region 8 along with Wyoming, Nebraska, Kansas, Iowa, and Missouri. These regions are important when it comes to organ allocation because, "with the exception of perfectly matched donor kidneys, organs are offered to sick patients within the area in which they were donated before being offered to other parts of the country."[1] This policy helps to lessen organ preservation time, reduce costs, and increase access to transplantation.

So multiple state laws, federal laws, and regional considerations all determined how organs got allocated. Now, all that applied, of course, only to organs from deceased donors, cadaveric organs. The same regulatory scheme did not apply in live organ donation. However, the prohibitions against organ selling set out in NOTA and UAGA did apply, whether the organ came from a cadaver or from a live donor.

It was bewildering. The walls of the labyrinth were built of laws and regulations, but I was being driven through the twists and turns by medical imperatives. I was not yet required to ask the Really Big ethical questions. How far would I be willing to go to get myself a kidney? Would I be willing to pay for one? Even if it meant violating the laws of another country? I was too busy just staying alive, remaining determined to stay off dialysis, relying instead on a good diet and a stubborn sense of hope.

Still, the one question that never had to beg for attention was the family question. A lot of people have a very romantic picture of families uniting, pulling together as a single loving unit in times of medical emergency. But one of the bitter lessons I learned that fall and winter was this: In the real world, real people faced with the real, complex problems they must solve to make it through the maze do not always come up with the same answer. During the weeks before I had ever heard of the idea of going abroad to buy a kidney,

I was torn between equally bad alternatives. Do I wait for more than 3 years? Do I go on dialysis? Do I accept a donation from Gregg or someone else in my family?

These were gut-wrenching issues that tore our family in conflicting directions. We never really wavered in our love for each other. And I never really doubted that Cindy cared for me. But each of us had a different agenda. She adamantly opposed any of her sons giving me a kidney. I adamantly refused to go on dialysis.

The time spent waiting on the list ticked slowly by.

There had to be another alternative.

CHAPTER SEVEN

THE GLOBAL MARKETS
FOR ORGANS

For years, I had enjoyed the drive from my law firm's high-rise in downtown Denver to our suburban Cherry Hills home with its sweeping views of the Rockies. Usually I made the trip in twilight or darkness, and seeing the thousands of twinkling lights rising in the distance always comforted me. But by 2004, the home fires were raging at the Farber residence and my 20-minute drive home was filled with dread. Our three sons had moved out and were living on their own. There was no one to turn to when Cindy ambushed me at the front door. "Did you find a kidney today?"

"No," I said, and started to explain to her: There was a crisis at the office this morning and there were so many phone calls and meetings this afternoon. But I just let it drop and walked past her, down the long hallway and into the kitchen.

Cindy was walking behind me, muttering, "Great—just great! I suppose I'm going to have to end up giving you one of my kidneys. You sure as hell aren't going to take one from any one of my sons."

This scene was unfolding with greater frequency. It made me uncomfortable. I grabbed some leftovers from the refrigerator, threw them on a paper plate, zapped them in the microwave, and headed down to the media room in the basement. I hit "play" on my DVD player and lost myself in *Citizen Kane* for the umpteenth time.

What was it about the story of Charles Foster Kane that so compelled me? Just how much could I identify with a man of great wealth and power whose only weakness traced to his childhood? An hour into the drama, long before the mystery of Rosebud was solved for the audience, I was asleep in my leather recliner.

My physical, mental, and emotional resources were being depleted rapidly.

Cindy and I were circling each other like opposing lawyers in a capital case. She was furious that I hadn't figured out a way to get a kidney transplant without putting at risk the health of one of our sons, especially Gregg, who had tested as a perfect match. She was stressed out, maybe even more so than me, and she was unrelenting.

Cindy came from a very wealthy family. She was accustomed to seeing most problems dealt with through influence or money: the economic solution. She felt I should figure out a way to buy myself a kidney from the best possible source outside the immediate family. And I really couldn't blame her. In my heart, I agreed with her and shared her protective instincts. I certainly did not relish asking anyone—let alone my wife or one of my sons—to put his or her life in danger by giving me a kidney. And no amount of reassurance that the risk of kidney donation is actually fairly slight could stop me from thinking of it as "putting their lives in danger."

I felt isolated without Cindy to lean on or talk to. Instead, her dukes were always up. She reminded me every day that I solve other people's problems for a living. She had seen me work miracles for my clients.

Why was I suddenly so helpless in this situation?

Other long-standing issues were at play, of course. We all have our weak spots, and Cindy had difficulty dealing emotionally with family medical crises, particularly since she had lost her mother to cancer. Now, she had decided that she didn't want to talk to me until

I'd figured out how to get an organ. It didn't help that she was a donor candidate, too. Everyone in the family had been tested, and Cindy was a good three-antigen match. Still, we both knew that she was not emotionally suited to being a donor. Her misgivings about medical matters and her powerful maternal instincts made her insistent that none of our sons should do it, either.

Our two younger boys, Brad and Brent, had qualified as potential donors in preliminary blood tests, but since both Cindy and Gregg had tested so much higher, no further tests were done on them. Brad had volunteered to be the donor, but he was scheduled to begin law school at Yeshiva University in New York City that May. And Brent—our family's playboy—had his own misgivings.

But Gregg had stepped up to say that he would donate his kidney to me.

"I know I'm going to be the one who gives you a kidney," he often said.

I appreciated his willingness to volunteer, but I didn't want him to feel pressured. "Do you really want to do this?" I asked him one time.

Gregg was a newlywed at that point. He had just married a woman named Sara and they were planning to start their own family. He had plenty of reasons to beg off.

"Look, Dad," he said to me. "Nobody wants to have surgery or give up an organ, but if I can give you life that way, how could I not do it?"

I was struck by his honesty and clarity. I never doubted Gregg's willingness to be my donor. Still, I hesitated to ask him to make such a sacrifice for me. Fathers are not supposed to ask their sons to put their lives at risk for them. I was supposed to be his source of strength, not the other way around.

Then in February, what had been murky and abstract became clear and concrete.

Before then I had garnered only the vaguest awareness of the black market trade in transplant organs. But early in the month I was contacted by another Denver attorney, an acquaintance. She told me her husband, Sol (not his real name), had gone to Turkey to buy a kidney in late 2003. Sol had not been able to qualify for the transplant waiting list in the United States because he was considered a poor risk. He had waited for more than 3½ years before learning about Dr. Zaki Shapira, an Israeli surgeon, formerly the head of some big transplant program at some big hospital outside Tel Aviv.

Sol's wife told me that Dr. Shapira operated kidney transplant clinics in Turkey, Latvia, and South Africa. She told me that prior to Sol's transplant, the Israeli surgeon had assured him that his organ donor would be Jewish and Israeli.

"You get it from where you descended," Dr. Shapira had promised him.

Before his operation, Sol did meet his donor, she said, or the man represented to be his donor. The stranger spoke only Hebrew, no English, and, Sol admitted, he really had no way of knowing whether his kidney came from this man or some other person.

For all you know, it could have come from a camel, I thought while hearing this account of Sol's adventure. I was feeling pretty skeptical about the whole business.

To get his transplant done, Sol had traveled to Turkey, where he had checked into a hotel on the European side of Istanbul. The next morning a black limousine had picked him up and taken him to a clinic on the Asian side of the city. The transplant was done the next morning. After the surgery, he spent 5 days recuperating. The clinic and all of his accommodations were "spic-and-span," according to Sol.

It all sounded so neat and tidy. But I found it hard to swallow. Nothing went down that easy in the Middle East. I kept flashing back to that movie *Midnight Express*, where the young guy gets thrown in a Turkish prison to rot. Maybe it wasn't a true picture of the country, but it was enough to give me the willies.

Finally, I met with Sol and learned more. All of his postsurgery care was done back in Denver at Presbyterian/St. Luke's Medical Center. He said the staff there had had no problem with the fact that his transplant had been done in another country by an unknown doctor. Sol described Dr. Shapira as an older Israeli who worked closely with a Turkish assistant. I grilled him about them. He admitted he couldn't say for certain if Dr. Shapira had actually performed the transplant. It all seemed very sketchy to me, but Sol was happy with his results and he appeared to be doing well with his new kidney.

At the end of our discussion, Sol gave me the phone number for Dr. Shapira, but I put it aside for the time being. I needed to know more about this mysterious doctor and the entire process of shopping for an organ outside of the United States. I wasn't certain it was legal, ethical, or safe. And even if it was, it still didn't seem like a very appealing option.

After I spoke with Sol, a mutual friend offered to put me in touch with people in Israel who knew Dr. Shapira. I also heard from my brother-in-law, Jimmy Lustig, who, concerned about my welfare, had taken it upon himself to contact the doctor about my case.

Friends and family started pushing me toward Turkey, but the harder they pushed, the more I balked. Cindy suited up as head cheerleader for the Turkey team. She was relentless and she had backup. My friend and client Ken Tuchman, then chairman of the board of the global outsourcing company TeleTech Holdings, called once a week, offering to jump in his plane with me to go to Canada, India, or South America to see if there were other alternatives.

I had trouble approaching the purchase of a vital organ as if I were buying an exotic car or custom-tailored suit. Nobody seemed to get that I had very strong concerns about trusting these unknown doctors in some foreign land with my life. I had not done enough research to know if it was even legal for an American citizen to go to Turkey for an organ transplant, or for a doctor in Turkey to provide an organ and perform such an operation on an American citizen. And it didn't soothe my fears that Dr. Shapira and others on his staff had repeatedly instructed Sol to "keep this quiet."

I am paid to consider the worst-case scenarios for our clients and to protect them if something goes wrong with a business deal or a court case. I certainly didn't have to be the world's smartest lawyer to work up a long list of things that could go wrong in a secretive Turkish transplant clinic trading in human kidneys from dubious sources. Still, I had to check out this unappealing option, if for no other reason than to appease the increasingly vocal members of my wife's pro-Turkey team.

Finally, I put in a call to Dr. Shapira. When he came on the line, I introduced myself as a friend of Sol's from Denver and told him I needed a kidney transplant.

I sound like some scumbag trying to buy a pound of pot, I thought.

The doctor's next question did nothing to ease my mind.

"What religion are you?" he asked.

"What difference does that make?" I said.

His reply was immediate—and it matched what he had told Sol: "Because I like to get them from where they descended."

I told him I was Jewish. Without further comment or question, he stated his price: "One hundred thousand dollars US will cover everything, from start to finish."

No money down, no payments for 6 months! I thought.

The transplant could take place in as little as 3 weeks, he said. I would simply have to get to Turkey. He would make all the other arrangements. There was no talk about whether the cost of the organ was included in the $100,000. That was implicit.

I assumed the donor would be paid something for the kidney. I didn't want to think about other potential scenarios regarding that part of the deal.

My concern that I was being sucked into some dark skullduggery only heightened after the phone call, but I found myself shipping my medical records to Dr. Shapira as he had instructed. He phoned a few days after receiving them to discuss my medical history. I told him I had once had basal cell skin cancer, but I had been thoroughly tested to get on the US kidney waiting list, and there was no sign of cancer anywhere in me at the time. He said that would be no problem.

Then, before I could fully consider the next step, Dr. Shapira announced that my surgery was scheduled for May 16 in Istanbul. I said I would be there. I realized that my only other options were many years of being hooked to a dialysis machine, risking the health of my son and the wrath of my wife, or death. Not an appealing trio of choices.

Almost immediately word got out that I had decided to go to Turkey. I never knew who talked first. But this time, Dr. Igal Kam, the Denver transplant surgeon I had previously consulted, made no effort to hide his disapproval. He was an Israeli, like Zaki Shapira, and had crossed paths with the infamous "organ outlaw" on many occasions—as I was to learn in greater detail during our talks while I worked on this book. Still, at the time, his voice of dissent was all but drowned out by a group of five who announced they were going with me to Istanbul for the surgery. They made it sound like a luxury voyage: the Kidney Cruise! Fun for the whole family!

Team Turkey consisted of Cindy, Jimmy Lustig, Jim and Lynne Sullivan, and Lee Alpert. They were packed before I could say "Istanbul." I felt their caring, but it was like being swept up in their plan for my life. I resisted, but my resistance was fading.

Then Dr. Shapira called again, with orders to send his payment in advance. That bothered me. I didn't want to be rushed. I needed to do more research. Late the next night, when Cindy was asleep, I went to my study and booted up my computer. Thanks to Google, I was on Dr. Shapira's Web site in seconds. It was chilling:[1]

If you are suffering from end-stage Kidney Disease, and need Kidney Transplantation, we can help. Our Team coordinates Organ Transplantation at leading Transplant Centers in the world. The Medical staff of our organization includes surgeons, nephrologists, cardiologists and anesthetists, all specialized in Transplantation Medicine and surgery [and] responsible [for] up to date medical evaluation of patients and donors and their appropriate matching. This medical team, headed by Prof. Zaki Shapira (with experience of more than 2000 kidney transplantations), accompanies you all the way: evaluation, surgery, recovery and long-term follow-up. The logistic team is responsible for all the legal and monetary administration with the chosen Center as well as for the Transportation to the Center and back for patients and their . . . family members. *In case of graft failure during the first six months after the transplantation, the company will provide a second Transplant on her own expenses.* [emphasis added]

Forget the quirky English translation. What really struck me was that Dr. Shapira was brazenly offering his two-for-one guarantee like some fake-gem salesman on the Home Shopping Network. Then and there, I vowed to check him out more thoroughly before packing a single sock. For hours that night and for several weeks afterward, I devoted any time I could spare to learning as much as I could about Dr. Shapira and the murky world of human organ markets.

I shared my concerns with Lynne Sullivan, who'd become my

medical advocate. As always, she stepped up to help with the research. She was dogged in her pursuit of knowledge, both on and off the Internet.

"So," said Lynne, "you fly to Istanbul and check in to some hotel. The next day a car comes and takes you away. Your family and friends are not allowed to go along. They must stay in the hotel the whole time. You are taken to a clinic where there is no visitation. You're there for 7 days. Steven, this just doesn't work. You have to learn a lot more about it." Soon my eye-opening education began.

I learned fairly quickly that I had every reason to be cautious about Dr. Shapira and the international organ transplant scene. In October 1996, the *Jerusalem Post* reported that the Israeli government had banned the country's leading kidney transplant surgeon— the very same Zaki Shapira—from performing transplants using organs from live donors.[2] He was then head of the kidney transplantation unit at the Rabin Medical Center Beilinson Campus in Petach Tikva, near Tel Aviv. The newspaper story claimed that a government committee had uncovered "strong evidence" that Dr. Shapira had violated regulations prohibiting the transfer of organs from live donors to unrelated recipients. While no criminal charges were brought against him at that time, the police had launched an investigation.

The *Post* said poor Palestinians had been selling their kidneys and Dr. Shapira had been transplanting them into wealthy Israelis and foreigners. But the article admitted that it had no real proof the surgeon had actually taken money for this. The story said that while a medical committee had questioned whether Dr. Shapira was properly following the ethical codes, its members also had had difficulty substantiating claims against him.

Israel at the time had no explicit criminal laws governing the use of donated organs or forbidding their sale, but health ministry regulations prohibited a person from giving an organ to anyone who was not a first-degree relative, according to the *Post* story. It also noted that Dr. Shapira had admitted in a hearing that he had not always followed official ministry rules on checking donors' credentials. He claimed he had acted in such cases solely from "altruism in an effort to promote transplants at all costs."

That story was one of several sources that called into question Dr. Shapira's practices without condemning him outright. Others were far less tolerant. In 2001, Dr. Nancy Scheper-Hughes, the head of the investigative watchdog group Organs Watch, issued a statement calling Dr. Shapira "a transplant outlaw" and alleging that since the early 1990s he had used Arab brokers to locate willing kidney sellers among poor Palestinian workers in the Gaza Strip and West Bank.

Dr. Scheper-Hughes reported that when the outlaw came under fire in his native land, he simply moved his transplant practice to Turkey and other Eastern European countries "where the considerable economic chaos of the past decade has created parallel markets in bodies for sex and for kidneys."[3] In her report, the anthropologist told of a Shapira patient named Mr. Tati, a former heart attack victim who could not get on the regular transplant list. Minutes after receiving a kidney allegedly purchased from an Iraqi soldier, Organs Watch claimed, he had another heart attack that was followed by kidney rejection, and he was "returned home close to death." That report did wonders for my confidence in Dr. Shapira.

While most of the information Lynne and I dug up on him seemed to be damning, we also found testimonials from former patients who loudly sang his praises. A report on ArabicNews.com described in glowing terms an unusual "kidney swap" Dr. Shapira performed in Tel Aviv.[4] In this case, the wife of a Jewish man from Jerusalem with kidney malfunction couldn't donate her kidney to him because she was not a match. At the same time, an Arab from a village near Haifa was not a match for his wife, who was suffering from kidney damage. Apparently, Dr. Shapira figured out that the Jewish guy's wife was a good match for the Arab guy's wife and the Arab husband was a good match for the Jewish one. He supervised the back-to-back transplants and was lauded for it in that account.

Then, later in 2001, the *New York Times* quoted Dr. Michael Friedlaender from Hadassah University Hospital as stating: "'Shapira is a mastermind. . . . He's made a big business out of this. I'm revolted by the amount of money he's making, but not by what he's doing. He's helped a lot of patients.'"[5] The *Times* also quoted a lawyer who said Dr. Shapira "'doesn't feel as though he is bound by national laws if these laws do not suit him. He arrived at the conclusion that if he didn't do something to stop people from dying on dialysis, then nobody would.'" It was unclear just what laws Dr. Shapira might have broken or where he might be subject to jurisdiction, the lawyer said.

An Israeli official told the reporter that there were suspicions about Dr. Shapira's activities, but no one had been able to prove that he'd done anything illegal. "'The patients won't testify because he's saved their lives. . . . I think Dr. Shapira should be brought to trial, but I'll bet he never will be,'" the Israeli official said. "'Sometimes it seems to me that transplantation is as much a moral failure as it is a medical success.'"

The controversies over Dr. Zaki Shapira's purchase and sale of organs led our investigation into the scary underworld of the international organ markets that were thriving around the world. I began to see vaguely what I now see clearly: The markets for organs were thriving because of the three great forces that drive today's events: economics, and especially globalization, spreading free markets and the "commodification" of flesh both living and dead; politics, especially the forces of sovereignty in its various modern forms; and laws, especially the expansion of the personal right of self-autonomy and limits on the authority of the state.

In the late 1990s, Organs Watch delved deeply into the origins of this underworld. Dr. Scheper-Hughes first traveled to Latin America to track down rumors of organ stealing that began in Brazil and Guatemala in the 1980s and then spread to other regions and countries. She also reported that questionable practices were commonplace in South Africa both during and after the apartheid government. In that country, she said, organ transplant practices revealed "the marked social and economic cleavages that separate donors and recipients into two opposed and antagonistic populations."[6]

Loopholes in South Africa's 1983 Human Tissue Act allow "appropriate" officials to practice a form of "presumed consent."[7] If, after reasonable attempts to do so, they cannot locate the potential donor's next of kin within the period of time when organ retrieval is possible, they can presume consent and harvest a deceased's organs. In 1997, a South African court refused to create a universal right to dialysis and kidney transplants because of the nation's limited resources. As a result, commercialism expanded. "In the absence of a national policy regulating transplant surgery, and of any regional, let alone national, official waiting lists, the distribution of transplantable organs is informal and subject to corruption."[8]

A *New York Times* investigation found a case connecting the organ trade in Brazil with that in South Africa.[9] A Brazilian named Alberty José da Silva arranged with an Israeli organ broker named Ilan Peri to sell his kidney to an American woman in a transplant that took place in South Africa. The *Christian Science Monitor* uncovered a strangely similar story in which another Brazilian went to the same hospital in South Africa, where he sold a kidney to an Israeli.[10] Investigators tracked the transaction and it helped lead to a major bust in December 2003, when police in both countries arrested 14 people on charges of illegal organ trafficking.

The *Monitor* noted that buying and selling kidneys across three continents "is, in some ways, the perfect 21st-century crime. . . . [I]t occurs in several jurisdictions, all of which are thousands of miles apart. And it's hard to determine where exactly the crime—handing over the money—takes place. And if one country starts cracking down, the syndicate can hop to another."

The troubling information Lynne and I dug up on the organ markets in Latin America and South Africa seemed mild compared to what we learned about their Asian counterparts. In Thailand, according to one study of Far East practices, despite "the objection of medical and legal authorities, many doctors have illegally arranged for their patients to pay fellow Thais for their relatives' kidneys. As in all other Asian countries, families in Thailand are unwilling to donate an organ from a deceased relative."[11] But a lot of traffic deaths occur in that country, and a lot of hospitals have begun to promote themselves as centers for "medical tourism" specializing in procedures ranging from cosmetic surgery to organ transplantation. "Selling organs," says the study, "can be highly profitable. . . . [T]he weaknesses in Thailand's regulatory efforts are flagrant. . . . They let misdeeds occur."

In the Philippines, I learned that kidney disease has a very special history because President Ferdinand Marcos suffered from it.[12] During his 21-year rule, Marcos underwent two kidney transplants. He established the National Kidney and Transplant Institute, which, according to the same study, became the "leading public transplant center in the country, performing more transplants than any other hospital, public or private." And where do all those kidneys come from? "In fact, they are sold openly and legally." Doctors and state officials readily defend sales of kidneys, citing the views of "ethicists" who argue that selling one's organs is a matter of free choice. And when asked whether most transplant recipients were among the elite, those who were able to afford the purchase of a kidney and the associated lifelong costs, the response was, yes, this is true, but the Philippines is "a very poor country."

Today the Philippines is one of the top five organ-trafficking hot spots according to a 2007 World Health Organization (WHO) report.[13] On the Internet, photos show men from the notorious Manila slum known as One-Kidney Island raising their shirts and arms to display the scars on their sides, marking where the kidneys they sold had been removed.[14] Web sites for private clinics like the Beverly Hills Medical Group, which operates facilities in Manila, advertise openly with detail and subtlety.[15]

When I was doing my research with Lynne, the most disturbing reports of all came from China, where the organs of executed prisoners were being sold.[16] The Chinese government denied it, but the Internet was swarming with graphic photos and first-person accounts documenting it. One Web site offered testimony from Thomas Diflo, MD, the director of renal transplantation at the New York University Medical Center. He noted that several of his patients were Chinese-Americans who had just returned from their native country with new kidneys. Several admitted they had received their kidneys from executed prisoners.

China at the time classified more than 68 crimes as capital offenses, including, under some circumstances, car theft, embezzlement, and the discharging of a firearm, according to Dr. Diflo's account and others in the media. Each year, the number of executions in China exceeded by at least twofold the total number of executions in the rest of the world combined. Official government figures at the time put the number of executions at around 5,000 annually, but nongovernmental sources estimated the actual number to be more than twice that. Of this figure, it was estimated that 1,600 executed prisoners would donate some 3,200 organs annually, according to Dr. Diflo.

At the time, China concocted various fictions to cover its organ-selling activities, according to human rights activists. It claimed that it had the consent of the prisoner in many cases and the consent of the family in others, as well as that the family had failed to collect the body in others. Still, many accounts contended that organs often were taken before the prisoners were even dead, because "fresher is better" in the organ business. Some even reported that the Chinese used "death vans" that drove up to the prisons and executed the prisoners on the spot so their organs could be taken "fresh."

Since I had my transplant, China has passed laws against organ trafficking. Some say that, nevertheless, the practice still flourishes. The issue is one of detection and enforcement.

And as horrifying as the Chinese practices sounded, I learned that India has the world's oldest, best established, and most studied market for buying and selling organs, especially kidneys from live donors. Dr. Scheper-Hughes began writing about India's "organs bazaars" in the 1980s, describing flourishing markets in the slums of Mumbai, Calcutta, and Madras.[17] But her writing was based on reports that appeared in the country's weekly periodicals and in several special reports produced by ABC and the BBC. It was unclear at the time how much of this reporting could be trusted. Then, in the early 1990s, more-scientific articles began to confirm these reports.

Dr. Scheper-Hughes has stated that the first rumblings of a commercial market in human transplant organs appeared in 1983, when an American doctor, H. Barry Jacobs, established the International Kidney Exchange in an attempt to broker the purchase of kidneys from living donors in Third World countries, especially India. By the early 1990s, living donors were involved in roughly 2,000 kidney transplants being performed each year in India.

The Indian market in kidneys, which catered largely to wealthy patients from the Middle East, was forced underground after the passage of a new law in 1994 that criminalized organ sales. Weak enforcement, however, led to the growth of an even larger black market in kidneys, one controlled by organized crime figures associated with the global heroin markets, according to Dr. Scheper-Hughes.

By the time I was conducting my research, India had become known as the "great organ bazaar" and the "warehouse for kidneys."[18] One study said that when the government began clamping down on the organ trade inside the country, the market makers simply began exporting their wares. There were reports of "kidney tours" in January 1995, in which racketeers lured 1,000 poor Indian donors abroad for removal of their kidneys for transplanting.

India had so many illicit sales of kidneys, in fact, that statistical reporting on the aftereffects became possible. The *Journal of the American Medical Association* in 2002 reported on 305 people in southern India who had sold their kidneys. It compared their economic and health statuses before and after their surgeries: "The income of the sellers declined by one-third after selling a kidney and nearly all had a worsening of their health." The vast majority of sellers had sold their kidneys to pay off debts, and 95 percent said that a desire to help a sick person with kidney disease was not really a factor in their decision to sell. Fifty-four percent had been below the poverty line at the time of the sale, but by the time of the follow-up interview, their statuses had declined even more dramatically, so that 71 percent were below the poverty line. Eighty-six percent of the sellers reported a worsening of their overall health, according to the study.

While the debates raged in India, the organ markets grew. In January 2004, the *Hindu* featured a study that concluded: "Commerce in kidneys has been increasing over the years in the country, in spite of the enactment of a law to regulate it. Ironically, the level of commercial exploitation in organ transplants appears to have increased" since the passage of the 1994 law. It was clear that poverty was "driving the sale of organs" and current laws were inadequate to stop it, the article said. It also said that possible reasons for the rise in commerce in organs included weak cadaveric organ transplant programs, the absence of an organ registry at the national or state level, and poorly developed brain death certification procedures. Yet many countries have weak transplant programs, nonexistent or poorly organized donor registries, and uncertain brain death procedures and still do not necessarily host underground markets for transplant organs.

As recently as January 2008, CNN ran videos of poor Indian workers who claimed to have been kidnapped and robbed of their kidneys—without even being paid for them![19] The workers had been found lying on cots, receiving no medical care. Like the men from One-Kidney Island, they pulled their pajama shirts up so their lurid fresh scars could be seen by the world. The doctors who later examined these workers reported that the operations that had removed their kidneys had been performed very professionally.

Urban legend had become graphically real. The Indian press went wild.

A week later, the mastermind of the ring, Amit "Dr. Horror" Kumar, age 40, was arrested in Nepal with $230,000 in cash and a check for $24,000 in his pockets. Nepal promptly extradited him to India, where the authorities paraded him before the television cameras. Dr. Horror appeared defiant, a scarf jauntily wrapped around his neck, his eyes hooded, his lips snarling. The *New York Times* reported that "several kidney rings have been exposed in India in recent years, [but] the police said the scale of this one was unprecedented. Four doctors, five nurses, 20 paramedics, three private hospitals, 10 pathology clinics and five diagnostic centers were involved."[20]

Under existing Indian law, only a recipient's spouse, parents, brother, or sister can donate, and organ selling is illegal. So again the problem is one of detection and enforcement. When India began cracking down on its organ trade, the markets simply shrugged and migrated across the border to Pakistan, which in 2007 replaced India on the WHO list of the top five organ-selling countries, along with China, the Philippines, Egypt, and Colombia.[21]

No one knows for certain why India became the original epicenter for illicit organ markets in the 1980s and 1990s. It may have been due to a lack of regulations and enforcement, though many countries have that problem. Poverty and overpopulation probably also played an important role. Whatever the causes, the organ markets in India spawned imitators abroad. And while the organ trade has stayed active in the country of its origin, its epicenter seemed to have shifted, at the time of my research, to the Middle East.

It was inevitable, I suppose, that the growing trade in organs in the Middle East would become infused with the volatile politics of the region. My research with Lynne took us to a Seattle-based Web site called Voices of Palestine that posted a letter to CanWest Global Communications Corporation head Israel Asper, asking him why Asper's newspapers, unlike other media outlets, hadn't published accounts of possible Israeli theft of organs from nonnationals who had died in the country. The letter cited these cases under headlines like[22]

Was a Ukrainian Murdered That a Jew Might Live?

Was a Scotsman Murdered That a Jew Might Live?

Three Palestinian Teenagers Murdered by Born-to-Kill Jews, Then Stripped of Organs

An Organ Robbery in Beersheba

Israel Is Deep into Organ Trafficking

And just think of the propaganda value of the big bust in Istanbul that netted the infamous organ outlaw, Zaki Shapira, in April

2007! Ironically, several months later, the Turkish courts freed Dr. Shapira for a "lack of prosecutable evidence." I can't help but wonder about what really went on behind the scenes of that *Midnight Express* scenario.

Still, perhaps the most ironic thing I've learned is this: While political controversy swirls around the role of Israelis in the global organ trade, it is the sworn enemy of Israel—the Islamic Republic of Iran—that plays a unique role in the global markets for organs.[23] On the one hand, Iran's theocratic government outlaws the use of organs from cadavers because, according to strict fundamentalist doctrine, that could violate the strictures of the Koran. But on the other hand, the Iranian government actively sponsors an open market for live kidneys. That's right. While countries like Pakistan and the Philippines allow sales of organs, only in Iran is the kidney trade fully legalized, fully regulated, and fully organized. Indeed, it is operated by two government-endorsed organizations. One puts possible recipients and donors in touch with each other and organizes medical tests to ensure compatibility, while the other pays the donor about $15,000 from government funds.

The Iranian system has virtually eliminated kidney waiting lists, says one study. An official boasted that it was a "new chapter in the world's transplantation history" and "an innovation in the Islamic Republic." Still, the study found that 90 percent of the sellers of kidneys complained of impaired physical ability and ill health after their surgeries, 70 percent suffered from depression, and 60 percent suffered anxiety. Several said they had attempted suicide or knew of donors who had killed themselves. Seventy percent reported feeling "worthless" after the operation and 85 percent said, if given the chance to go back and do it over again, they would not sell their kidneys and would advise others against doing so. Many spoke of social rejection and marital conflict after selling their kidneys.

These are disappointing statistics coming from a country where the organ trade is legal and regulated. Some say this is inevitable at the beginning of any social experiment. Take the life insurance business as an example. A hundred years ago, many in society were repelled and disgusted by the thought of buying life insurance, viewing it as a wager on the life of a loved one that turned death into a commodity. There are those who believe that society will one day come to accept the trade in human organs for transplantation in much the same way that we have come to accept life insurance. They claim that it will evolve into a legal, efficient, humane, and properly regulated market. But others are not so sure.[24]

As things stand today in America, if your heart, lungs, kidneys, or liver fails, you will likely die unless you get a transplant. If you can afford it, you can go abroad to buy an organ. The WHO makes it easy for you. Its 2007 report on the state of the international organ trade bemoans "the paucity of scientific research," then lists eight Web sites for transplant tourism, three in China, four in Pakistan, and one in the Philippines.[25] It even lists the prices of various "transplant packages" that are available. A new kidney from Liver4You in Manila, for example, would cost you $85,000.

The WHO report does not mention Zaki Shapira's Web site, which described his operations to me 4 years ago. Nor does it include Beautiphil Health Holidays, the Beverly Hills Medical Group, or Health Tours India, with its fetching "Life Smile Health Care." There are so many choices available today.

But suppose you can't afford to go abroad to buy an organ or you choose not to do so out of concerns over ethics, legality, or safety. You have to stay in America.

If you are unable to get an organ through the official registries and waiting lists, you can't just go out and buy one—legally. There is no free market in organs in America, but there is what some economists have called a "volunteer market."[26] In this "market"—loose, unorganized, and inconsistent across geographies and demographics—donors agree to give away their usable organs upon their deaths, or living donors agree to give up organs or portions of organs, usually to family members or someone they care about. In truth, this so-called "volunteer market" is just a fancy name for altruism.

Meanwhile, revolutionary strides in transplant surgery have led to an explosion in the demand for healthy organs. The *New York Times* reported that in 2005, more than 16,000 kidney transplants were performed in the United States, an increase of 45 percent over 10 years.[27] Moreover, during that same period, the number of people on the kidney waiting list rose by 119 percent, the story said. In other words, even though more people than ever are donating their organs, medical advances in surgery and the creation of better immunosuppressive drugs with fewer side effects actually increase the pool of good candidates for transplants, thereby making the spread between supply and demand grow even wider. Today, more than 6,500 people die in America each year while waiting for a kidney or other organ transplant.

This situation has created what some economists have described as a "basic supply-and-demand gap with tragic consequences."[28] We have to ask: How can the supply of human organs be increased to meet the demand for those who will die if they don't get a transplant? In the United States, organ donors have to "opt in" by signing on to a registry, but in Brazil and many European countries, it is just the opposite: Unless you or your family members affirmatively decline, your organs are harvested when you die. Even so, Europe still has a significant shortage of organs available for transplant. European medical communities struggle to figure out why.

And abuses are common in Brazil.[29] Since 1998 Brazil has had an "opt-out" presumed consent law, and that law has simply moved the problem from rumored organ stealing to abuses within the system. These abuses, according to Dr. Scheper-Hughes and others who have studied the problem, include organ sales, organ thefts, falsification of death certificates, and corruption in the distribution of organs. Since Brazil performs more than 12 percent of the kidney transplants in the world, this becomes a significant problem, both in absolute and relative terms.

One account states that the director of Rio de Janeiro's state morgue "welcomed the new law of presumed consent as a thoroughly modern institution which offered an opportunity to educate the 'ignorant masses' in the new democracy. But to the proverbial man and woman on the street . . . the new law is just another bureaucratic assault on their bodies. The only way to exempt oneself was to request new identity cards or driver's licenses officially stamped 'I am not a donor of organs or tissues.'"[30]

Would a presumed consent system work here in America? Recently, British prime minister Gordon Brown called for movement toward a presumed consent system in his country.[31] Chapters Eleven and Twelve discuss this alternative to our present system.

For now, however, it is clear. All you have to do is follow *Freakonomics* on the *New York Times*'s Web site. From a purely economic perspective, it makes perfect sense to eliminate the ban on selling human organs for transplant purposes here in America. The arguments are especially persuasive when it comes to kidneys, since most people can live safely with just one, and for livers, too, since small portions can now be regenerated into viable new organs. Some economists even contend that financial incentives would increase the supply of organs enough to eliminate the waiting lists altogether without materially increasing the total cost of transplant surgery.

But this is not pure economics. There are strong moral and ethical objections to the commodification of body parts, even in a time when it has become common to sell human sperm and eggs and to pay surrogate mothers. Class issues are involved. There are fears that desperate or chronically poor people will sell their organs just to survive or that they will become pawns of unscrupulous organ traders.

My research suggested that one day there might well be some form of legalized and regulated market for transplant organs in America, but it certainly would not develop in time for me. I had to find another way in the here and now.

I had done my due diligence. I had learned a lot. Many of my original assumptions had been challenged. I had to admit it was a very complex problem.

Still, the fact remained that I faced a difficult decision given the harsh realities. My choices were still limited. I could ask Gregg to donate a kidney to me and face the family upheaval that would inevitably ensue. I could roll the dice and pay Dr. Zaki Shapira for a kidney from an unknown source. Or I could go on dialysis.

Time was running out for me. My health was deteriorating.

I had to make a decision.

CHAPTER EIGHT

FINAL OPTIONS

From the time I first learned of Dr. Zaki Shapira until late April, while Lynne and I were researching those murky black markets and all the people around me were wringing their hands, my kidneys continued to fail. I felt a terrible weakness, a heavy sort of fatigue, and a loss of focus. My life was in grave danger and my options refused to change: a kidney from Gregg, Dr. Shapira's shady transplant operation in Turkey, dialysis—or death.

I was increasingly inclined to accept Gregg's offer, but because of Cindy's strident opposition, that option was becoming a serious threat if not to his health, then at least to family harmony. And while very few live kidney donors in the United States suffer adverse medical effects from the transplant surgery or life with one kidney, it is not entirely unheard of. What if Gregg's health took a turn for the worse because he donated his kidney to me? I did not on any level want to face that outcome.

So I passively allowed Team Turkey to make its plans to take me to Istanbul for my May 16 date with Zaki Shapira. And as I continued to vacillate—it was my body, after all—everyone freely weighed in. Cindy had become the quarterback of the team, pushing relentlessly for the goal line according to her own agenda. She was supported at that position by our brother-in-law, Jimmy Lustig, the halfback of the team.

Jimmy is married to Cindy's sister. He was the guy who had originally contacted Dr. Shapira on my behalf, without my even knowing about it. Jimmy kept trying to be helpful, but to me it felt somewhat intrusive. I was already overwhelmed with other people's interests. I didn't need to be juggling any more. "Steve closed himself off a bit to other people," says Jimmy, recalling those days. "He wasn't very receptive to my help. I thought that it was important that both sides—his side and Gregg's, both of their interests—be included to a greater degree in the family's decision-making process. But I wasn't really successful."

And sadly, says Jimmy, "To some extent, Steve put himself on that island of his."

Now, Jimmy was not the only character who saw things differently than I did. Brent, my middle son, recalls the reasons Gregg was the obvious chosen one, the right one to do the right thing and donate his kidney to me. Brent says he and Gregg and Brad talked many times about my situation. At first, he says, it was all tentative and abstract. The question—which of the three should donate his kidney—wasn't immediate or threatening. Then it turned scary. My condition deteriorated.

Each of my sons had been tested to determine his blood type. Brent knew nothing about the transplant process, so he talked to Denver doctors Mark Linkow, MD, and Rick Abrams, MD, and felt a little better after learning more about the low risks of donation. Still, Brent admits that he was afraid. "Whenever I thought about donating my kidney, I got nausea in my stomach," he recalls. "It was a very scary feeling for me. Whenever I thought about my dad and his life, of course, it made it a lot easier. But there were so many unknowns."

The turning point came, according to Brent, during one particular conversation. It was sometime in the middle of the day. Brad was still at college in Arizona and Gregg was living in Denver. Brent recalls that he was in his shirt sleeves, his collar open—"I never had to wear a tie"—at his office on the fourth floor of the Five-Seventy-Five Building at 51st and Lexington in Manhattan, working as a money manager.

All three of my sons were deeply concerned.

"Mom was becoming increasingly agitated," says Brent. "You would talk to her and she just couldn't talk about anything else. It had overtaken everything. She just kept saying, over and over, 'I'm going to do it before any of you are!' But all three of us knew we couldn't allow that to happen. She never would have recovered."

He does not mean medically. He means: "My mom and her family find it hard to cope with things, to get over things, to deal with things." So my sons had another of their continuing talks with neither of their parents on the line. Each repeated that he would be the donor if it came to that, but something about this conversation was different.

My sons were making their own decision. It was one they had hoped they could avoid. But when the time came and they felt they could wait no longer, it was not a matter of Brad's starting law school or Brent's fear of the surgery. It was simply a matter of blood type. All three had been tested, and Brad and Brent were both universal donors with an O-positive blood type. But Gregg had a blood type of A-negative. They had all known this for weeks, but they could no longer ignore its import.

"Gregg's blood type was the same as Dad's," says Brent. "So when we talked about it, at that point, it just all made sense. I mean, Gregg's blood type was a perfect match and ours wasn't. That meant Brad and I wouldn't be perfect six-point antigen matches, either, and as it turned out, Gregg would. So it was perfectly logical. All the pointers, the arrows, turned toward him. Gregg was the oldest and had always been the one to take the first step. He was the first to get fully tested and first to initiate all the phone calls. He was the one who always took the lead. At the end of that phone call, no stated decision had been made. But that was when we all knew Gregg would be the one."

After that, Brent was wracked with guilt. He talked to his brothers about it, insisting that he did not want Gregg to be the donor. He would ask, "Why him and not me?" Brad and Gregg assured him that they saw things the way they had already decided.

And now, in hindsight, Brent agrees, "It had to be Gregg all along. It was, like, his fate. We knew he would be the best because he was the strongest of the three of us. Physically and mentally, he was the right one."

Then, flashing forward, Brent adds, "No one in my family shows emotions. They never have. But on the morning of the transplant, seeing my dad and Gregg lying next to each other right before the surgery, I felt emotions come over me like I'd never felt before. I had never before expressed myself so much. And I've never cried so much. I probably had never told Gregg that I loved him before. But on that day I went over to him lying there and kissed him on the forehead and told him that I loved him."

So Cindy and Jimmy were pushing for Turkey while my boys had made up their own minds. And then there was my good friend Jim Sullivan. When the idea of going to Turkey surfaced in February 2004, Jim thought it made perfect sense. He looks at things very simply: Got a leaky pipe? Call a plumber.

"Let's go," he would say to me, "and get it over with."

"What would you do?" I would respond.

"Probably," Jim would say, "I would get in my Ferrari and drive off a mountain in some sort of drama—but I'm not you."

Jim became Cindy's linebacker. She was intensely protective of Gregg, and she wanted me to go to Turkey to buy that kidney. To her and Jim, the economic solution was better than the emotional one. They saw it as the only option that made any sense. There was fierce debate among the Farbers and the Sullivans.

Whenever I would say "I don't want to die in Turkey," Jim would say that he—the protector and enforcer—would go with me to make sure I got out safely.

"I'll bring him home," Jim would say, sounding like the Vietnam vet that he is. To him, it was all about taking death into your own hands. The money solution was not really about money. It was about self-autonomy. Jim believes poor people die more gracefully than rich people. They do not have as many options. He says, "What's so simple for the poor is so difficult for those with privilege. That's the real difference between the haves and the have-nots. The have-nots are resigned to their fate. They do what they must do. They have so few false hopes."

In hindsight, Jim says that he was there not only to bring me home, but also to keep me grounded. He meant to repay the debt he owed me for what I had done for him during his dark days of bankruptcy.

Jim likes to tell this story, which he says perfectly describes our differing attitudes toward fear and death: "It was before Steve's illness had been revealed. We were coming back from a guys' weekend in Las Vegas. At the time, I was shopping for a company plane and we had rented a Learjet to take us back to Denver so I could see what it was like. We were playing rummy in the seats behind the cabin. Over Grand Junction we heard and felt a bump and a jolt. I went up to the cabin and asked the pilot what was going on. He pointed at his instrument cluster and said, 'Look, we've lost our hydraulics. I don't know if the wheels went down. If they didn't, we have no brakes.'"

"Have you dealt with this sort of thing before?" Jim asked the pilot.

"I've got no actual experience with it, but it happened to me once in a simulator."

"How'd you do?"

"We landed safely," said the pilot. "Look, this is a real emergency, so go back there and strap yourself in."

Jim went back to playing rummy with me. He did not tell me what was going on, but he did suggest that we strap ourselves in because it could get pretty bumpy going over the mountains. And it did get bumpy, so we put away our cards, put the tray table up, and pulled our seat belts tighter. When Centennial Airport, just south of Denver, finally came into view, I could see that emergency vehicles were waiting on the runway.

"I wonder who those are for?" I asked.

Jim looked sheepish and replied, "Well, uh, they're kind of for us."

The pilot landed smoothly. The landing gear had gone down, but the hydraulics were indeed shot, so the plane deployed its parachute to act as the backup for the brakes.

"Why didn't you tell me!" I demanded. I was furious.

Jim responded calmly, "Why worry about stuff you can't change?"

"But we could've died!" I said.

"Dying doesn't hurt," said Jim.

"Is that something you learned in Vietnam?" I asked.

"Yes, that's right," said Jim.

"Well," I said, "then how would you know? You didn't die in Vietnam."

Very few people know both me and Ernesto, the peasant and the power broker. One of them is Jim Sullivan, and I have heard him wax eloquent about Ernesto's story, about how it is the perfect example of how the haves and have-nots face death and hardship differently. Another is the woman who at the time was Jim's in-house counsel and business partner. Her name is Carolyn and she has known me for many years, both through her work with Jim and independently as a lawyer. As Jim's lawyer and a senior member of his management team, Carolyn also got to know Ernesto. She knew him as an employee of Jim's company and she drew up the legal papers that later helped Ernesto start his own business. She has met all his family. They have eaten at her home. She served them cheesecake from New York.

Carolyn thinks back to April 2004. Rumors were flying that I was going to Turkey to buy a kidney. And as Jim's confidant, she knew those rumors were true.

One day Ernesto came to see her. He was upright and straightforward. He told her he had learned a couple of years before that his sister had kidney disease and might someday need a transplant. After he was tested and learned he was a match, he began saving all his vacation time. He never took any time off, even if he or someone in his family was sick. He hoarded all that paid time off. Now, he needed to take it. His sister needed that transplant, and soon. He needed to donate his kidney to her.

It would only be for a few weeks, he said. The problem—unknown to Ernesto but clear to Carolyn—was that the company didn't let its employees accumulate paid vacation time from year to year. It was a use-it-or-lose-it system. Ernesto was entitled to far less paid time off than he realized. But in working with Ernesto, Carolyn had come to learn the story of his migration to America. She knew of his bravery in Guatemala and respected his hard work, his honesty, and his trustworthiness. She really liked him. So she didn't tell him that he couldn't have his time off with pay to donate his kidney to his sister. Instead, Carolyn said, "That's fine. Thanks for letting us know. You take all the time you need. You've earned it."

Ernesto said thanks and left her office. Carolyn immediately called Jim and told him what Ernesto had just said and how she had responded. She did not ask Jim for any sort of approval. She simply told him: The company would have to pay Ernesto for the time he had to take off. All of it. Whether it was within the rules or not.

Jim readily agreed. Ernesto was free to devote all of his attentions to saving Sandra's life—for the second time.

Near the end of April, about 3 weeks before I ended up getting my transplant from Gregg, I was eating Mexican food at the Blue Bonnet restaurant on South Broadway with my friends Debbie and Lee Alpert. At the table next to us sat a well-respected nephrologist who practiced at Rose Medical Center. I used to be the chairman of the board of trustees at Rose, so I knew most of the doctors who practiced there. This nephrologist, who was not my doctor, leaned over and asked me, "How are you feeling?"

"Okay," I answered, an automatic response, even though I had been feeling worse and worse—fatigued, weak, less energetic. By then, 7 months had passed since I had returned from Italy, and a full year had passed since I'd gone to that fund-raiser at the MacMillans' mansion.

The nephrologist looked me up and down. In a raised voice he said, "You just don't get it! You're near death! Have you ever seen the inside of a dialysis lab?"

"No," I said, and then I tried to blow him off. "I'm going to die someday. Does that mean I should go visit a cemetery?"

He refused to be shaken so easily. He said, "You're at the final hour. Get a transplant or get on dialysis immediately."

I felt like saying "Go screw yourself," but I usually don't talk that way, especially in public. And this was a very public confrontation in a very public place.

So instead of saying what I felt like saying, I drew a deep breath, kept my anger fully in check, and asked the nephrologist, "What would you do?"

He answered without hesitation: "Have your son give you one of his."

"But . . ."

"He has another."

"But . . ."

"Listen, you love your son, right?"

"Of course."

"And he loves you." The doctor lowered his voice. "So the worst possible thing for him is you dying. That way he won't have you."

Now, I resented this nephrologist at the time for having his confrontation with me in such an uncomfortable, public way. Still, he did make me think. I was close to going to Turkey to acquire what was said to be an Israeli kidney on the organ market. I even had my date to go there. Would I really show up for the surgery scheduled for May 16?

The next 3 weeks were very difficult for all of us. My options had not changed a bit: dialysis, death, Gregg, or Zaki Shapira. I had never wavered in my resolve to avoid dialysis. Nothing I had learned about it had ever changed my mind. And of course, death was not really an option. So I had to focus on Gregg and Shapira. They had become my last resorts.

I started to talk with Gregg and his wife, Sara, about Gregg's willingness to be my donor. I was struggling with that option, knowing all the while how much Cindy hated the idea, hated that it was even being considered. Throughout these discussions, Cindy was well aware of the way the winds were blowing, but she didn't really participate much, except to reaffirm, over and over again, her opposition to Gregg's donation.

Still, whether I liked it or not, I had to take a good, hard look at my oldest son. And whether he liked it or not, he had become my lifeline.

Gregg wore braces at age 32 to make himself even more perfect. He was tall and handsome and well built and athletic, clean-shaven like me, with some thinning of the dark hair on his high forehead, also like me. He had earned his undergraduate degree in business from the University of Colorado in Boulder and his master's in business from the University of Southern California. He was the sort of young man who knew he had led a privileged life, but would contend that it's not all it's cracked up to be.

Gregg says Cindy has always been very loving as a mother, but also exceedingly controlling. She's always trying to tell her sons what to wear, where to go, what to do. Gregg finds it hard to deal with. Well intentioned, it may be—he knows she does it only because she wants what is best for her sons—but still it has proved difficult for Gregg.

Early on, Gregg figured he would be the one to donate his kidney to me. He knew his mother would not be the donor. He also believed his middle brother, Brent, would not seriously consider it, though Brent had said he would. And his youngest brother, Brad, was just starting law school. In all fairness, Gregg thought, Brad could not be expected to step off his track, since Gregg already had gotten his education. Finally, Gregg knew that my sister would never donate to me since she and I have a distant relationship. I had no other siblings and my parents are both dead.

Pure and simple, by process of elimination, Gregg figured he would be the one—until the spring of 2004, when I told him, during a conversation at our family home, "There might be another option."

I described Sol's trip to Turkey to buy a kidney from Zaki Shapira. Gregg recalls, "Dad said he knew this guy who had done it, and it might be an option. And at the time I thought, *What a great idea!* Dad and I were both very interested in finding out more about this alternative. Was it really viable?"

We did not discuss the ethics much. I told him, "Look, you pay this amount and some of it goes to the donor and it's as much as the guy makes in a year, maybe more."

That made Gregg think. At first blush it seemed unethical, but he said to himself, *Wait a second! What if it was hair? You can buy and sell human hair. And it may be illegal here in America—but why? What's worse? That or Nike sweatshops in places like China and Mexico?* At that point, in his mind, his dad's survival overshadowed most issues.

But I was very concerned about the legalities and the ethics because I am a lawyer and my reputation is very important to me. I saw the ethical dilemmas—the possible exploitation of the poor—and I was not even sure whether what we were talking about was legal in Turkey.

I explained to Gregg that I had been told repeatedly, "You must understand you are not coming to Turkey for an organ transplant. You must deny that is your purpose if you are asked." This admonition strongly suggested that there was indeed some risk in going to a strange country for a kidney transplant, having the surgery there, and then having to get out again. What if something went wrong?

Gregg looked at the situation. His mother, Jimmy, Jim, and others were pushing hard for Team Turkey. Brent and Brad were beginning to lean that way, too. I was not moving up on the waiting list. Something had to be done.

But Gregg did not sign on. He began to question the idea of going to Turkey as soon as I began to explain the details as they unfolded according to my research. "Look," I said, "it worked for Sol, but we still don't know that much about it. There appears to be no board supervision of this practice in Turkey. And we don't know much about the safety of the procedure there or what their health care facilities are like."

"My dad," says Gregg, "portrayed the money side as just a matter of cost. It was going to cost $100,000, and $5,000 or $10,000—whatever—was going to go to the kid. That's what my dad called the donor: the kid. But he was really worried that something would go wrong, either on the health and safety side of things or on the legal side of things. He still wasn't sure it was legal in Turkey. And

I don't think he ever really found out, even though he has all these vast resources at his disposal."

Ultimately, I asked Gregg, "Can you imagine if this isn't legal and they find out? Would they try to keep me there? And if you went there with us, would they try to keep you there, too?" Visions of *Midnight Express* kept dancing in our heads.

At first, Gregg admits, when he heard me wonder out loud whether I could get safely in and out of Turkey, he thought to himself, *My dad is such a wuss.*

Then he remembered his first trip outside of the United States. It was 1994 and he was 22. He had just graduated from college. The prior December, it had rained constantly in Hawaii, so the family decided to take that year's winter vacation in Mexico. Nine people traveled together: Cindy and me with our three sons plus Jimmy and Debbie Lustig with their two kids. Gregg admits he was apprehensive. He had heard there was a lot of crime—"especially a lot of stealing"—in Mexico. And people said you had to be careful with the food and water. He had no idea what he was in for.

"We got to the airport at Los Cabos," he says, "and it was late morning. The nine of us must have had 20 bags or more—big suitcases—plus our golf clubs and all sorts of things. My mother always packs for a month even if she's only going for a week. Anyway, we did not know how things worked down there. We saw people were pushing a big button that lit a red or green light as they went through customs. If they got green, the customs people waved them through. We got red, of course."

The customs people did not wave our family through. Instead, they took us off to the side and opened all 20 of our suitcases. And just what did they find?

Gregg laughs, "It was shortly after Hanukkah, see, so a lot of what they found inside were new clothes—fancy, expensive designer labels—still in the original wrappings from the store.

Shirts still folded with pins inside plastic. Lots of clothes."

The customs people suspected we were bringing all those new clothes into the country for the purpose of starting a business without a permit or license. They simply could not imagine how any sane person could otherwise be bringing so many new clothes into the country—especially since we claimed we were coming into Mexico for only a short vacation. Soon we were being questioned by a young government functionary flanked by two police officers in blue uniforms. He was short and slight and they were big and bulky. He had black hair but no mustache, and he wore neither a uniform nor the Latin guayabera, but rather was dressed as a civilian in tan slacks and a white button-down shirt open at the neck, no tie. His official ID, encased in plastic, was clipped to his shirt.

Gregg smiles. "He was this little guy, five feet five at most, and pretty young, probably in his mid-twenties. And he was questioning us about all our new clothes."

"Where are you taking all these new clothes?" asked the government functionary.

"To the hotel," we insisted.

"Nobody brings this much for a vacation. How long are you planning to stay?"

"Two weeks."

"Why are so many of your clothes still in their wrappings?"

And so forth, until he said, "We think you are coming here to open a store."

"No, no!" shouted Gregg. At 22, he had something of a temper, which he claims he got from me. And, since he was big and strong, he wanted nothing more than to jump all over this dinky young government functionary.

I had to physically restrain him, he was so mad. "My dad," says Gregg, "had to hold me back. He said we could go to prison if I kept it up."

Finally the young functionary and his guards confiscated all of my family's luggage. They took our suitcases to a back room and left all of us standing there in the terminal. The entire confrontation had taken place right there, out in the open, in the terminal.

"At one point they came out," says Gregg, "and told us we could have our luggage if we gave them $40,000 in cash. My dad just laughed at them."

After an hour of waiting in the terminal, the family was going crazy. "Okay," said Gregg, "let's just get out of here and never come back."

"No," said the government people, "we can't let you leave the country."

So Cindy and her sister Debbie went with all the kids to the resort hotel where we were staying, leaving Jimmy and me behind at the airport to collect the luggage. It was by then about 11:00 in the morning on Christmas Eve.

At about 4:30 that afternoon, we showed up at the hotel—without the luggage.

I wiped my hand over my brow in a gesture my friends and family know well. Then I said, "I can't believe it. They won't listen to us, and they won't let us out."

I sighed deeply. This was supposed to be my vacation. Then I swung into action. I called former Denver mayor Federico Peña, who was then US secretary of transportation. I reached Federico in Albuquerque, where his father-in-law was the dean of the law school at the University of New Mexico. Federico said that he would call the White House. In the meantime, I should try calling his counterpart at the Mexican Transportation and Communications Ministry. His name was Jaimie Serra Puche, if I recall correctly, and he took my call without hesitation, even though it was Christmas Eve.

Next I called Tim Wirth, counselor at the State Department and a former senator from Colorado. Tim told me to call Jim Jones, the

American ambassador to Mexico. So I called Jones and caught him as he was on his way to church. I had talked to Jones before, since one of my younger partners, Cole Finnegan, had been chief of staff for him when he was a congressman from Oklahoma. Jones called his people at the American embassy and told them to call the young functionary at the airport and tell him the Farber family was perfectly okay, they should get their luggage back and be allowed to go in peace.

The reply from the government people at the airport was terse: "No! We don't take orders from the American ambassador. He's not our boss!"

So I called Tim Wirth back. By then it was 6:30 p.m. on Christmas Eve. Tim said he would call the White House. He also gave me the name and number of the woman he was going to call at the White House. I waited a little while and then called her. She said I did not need to call anymore. The White House already had heard from Secretary Peña and Senator Wirth. They would call the young government functionary at the airport and tell him the Farber family was perfectly okay, so please give them their luggage back and let them go on their way.

But when the White House called the airport at Los Cabos, it got the same answer: "No! We do not take orders from your White House. We only listen to our boss."

Finally, at about 7:30, as I was still working the phones, Jimmy Lustig returned to the airport, determined to return with those 20 suitcases of new clothes.

This time when the government functionary invoked his boss as the only one from whom he would take orders, Jimmy was ready for him. "Okay," he said, "just who is your boss? Where is your boss? I want to see him!"

By 9:00 p.m. on Christmas Eve, Jimmy was telling the young functionary's boss that someone from the White House of the president of the United States wanted to talk to him. Reluctantly, the boss took the call, only to hear what might be expected: Let the Farbers and their luggage go. These are people who know people in the highest of places!

And it was all true. Bill Clinton was in the White House at the time. A decade later, when he came to Denver to read his autobiography at the Tattered Cover Bookstore, I was the guy he called for a favor. I was the one who held the fund-raiser for the Clinton Library—and for countless other political and charitable causes—in my home in southeast Denver. The young functionary's boss got the message.

"Okay, fine," he said, "no problem."

By 10:30—roughly 12 hours after landing in Mexico—Jimmy had returned to the hotel with all 20 pieces of our luggage. Now, 12 hours of waiting, frustration, and hassle doesn't sound so awful

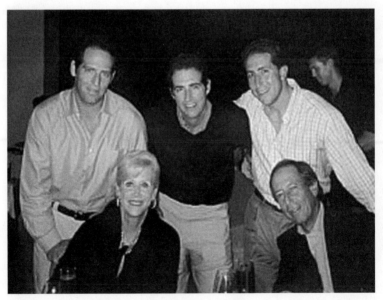

The Farber family on vacation in Hawaii, 2005.
Top row: Gregg, Brent, Brad. Bottom row: Cindy and Steve.

to simple folk like Ernesto Delaroca. He walked for that length of time each day when he journeyed back and forth between Guatemala and America. And his sister Sandra used to walk the 6 blocks to her dialysis center because there was simply no other way. They were poor. They did what they had to do, just like Jim Sullivan says.

But 12 hours seemed like an eternity to Gregg, the big, strong, hot-blooded son of the power broker. Today, Gregg admits he cannot conceive of walking to dialysis, let alone walking for 12 hours a day across rugged terrain to get to America. He says at the time, at that airport in Los Cabos, he simply wanted to pummel his tormentors, starting with that little government functionary.

This episode made a lasting impression on Gregg. It was 9 years before he again set foot inside Mexican borders.

So the leap in Gregg's mind from "what a wuss" to certainty took only an instant, once he recalled that Christmas Eve in the Third World. After all, if it took a call from the White House just to get your luggage through customs in Mexico, think about how much harder it would be to get his dad out of Turkey if something went wrong there. It may sound politically incorrect in hindsight, but it was all too real during the instant of that leap in Gregg's mind. And in that instant he knew that, after all was said and done, he would ultimately be the one who would donate his kidney to save my life. It had become inevitable.

"When finally my dad explained why he was worried—genuinely worried—about getting out of Turkey safely following the transplant," says Gregg, "at that exact moment I knew."

Despite the facts that growing up privileged was not all it is cracked up to be and that we had gone through our tumultuous times over the years, Gregg simply could not let me go to Turkey. The decision, in his mind, was made. It was a done deal.

He would donate his kidney to me.

He would end the madness that was consuming our family.

CHAPTER NINE

THE DAY OF OUR SURGERIES

The day before their surgeries, when Ernesto and Sandra were at the hospital to finish their final tests and start getting prepped, Sandra nearly backed out. She started crying uncontrollably. Ernesto says she was thinking too much about the anesthesia: "She was worried she would go to sleep and never wake up."

The nurse named Anita came and sat with them. Once more she talked them through all the risks of the surgery—and all the risks of not having it. Sandra realized that she had no choice. After about 30 minutes, she stopped crying and said okay. They were back on track. The waiting was almost over.

"Anita did everything for us," recalls Ernesto. "She stayed with us from the time we checked in until the surgery was over. In fact, Sandra did not actually meet the transplant surgeon"—Dr. Igal Kam—"until the day of the surgery."

Sandra and Ernesto went home after their final tests for their last night before surgery. Ernesto says he and Sandra were wearing identical plastic wrist bracelets that had both of their names on them. He was not nervous in the slightest. He was just ready to get it over with. It was all mental for him.

He and Sandra were told during their preadmission briefing not to eat or drink for at least 8 hours before the surgery. At 4:00 in the morning, everyone got out of bed and went to the hospital. They checked in and took Ernesto's weight one last time.

Neither he nor Sandra was afraid by then. All of their family—Gicela, Galilea, Edgar, and a couple of cousins—were there, as well as two American couples who worked with Amnesty International, Scott and Elena plus Bryan and Angela. Ernesto had met them several years before at a meeting of Amnesty International that was held at a church near Speer and Federal Boulevards in Denver's Spanish neighborhood. Both couples had just returned from working in Guatemala.

"I went to the church to talk to them about what was going on in Guatemala," says Ernesto, "and we became friends. Every couple of weeks we'd get together and have a picnic or dinner in one of our homes. They helped us a lot while Sandra was sick. They would drive her to her doctor's appointments when I couldn't because of work. They were always there for us."

Ernesto noticed that day that there were an awful lot of other people milling around in the hallways and the waiting rooms. He did not know someone important was having a kidney transplant that morning as well. He did not recognize any of the entourage of 30 that assembled as Gregg was giving his kidney to me.

Ernesto later learned that his boss's wife—Lynne Sullivan—had served trays of deli sandwiches to everyone in the waiting rooms that morning, the power broker's entourage and the Delaroca clan alike.

Mostly during those last 3 hours before he was wheeled into the operating room, Ernesto recalls feeling glad, relieved, "good with all these people around me. There was a lot of love in those waiting rooms," he says. When finally it was his and Sandra's turn, the family gathered around them and hugged them and said their good-byes. Ernesto was out by the time they wheeled him away. The last face he saw was his daughter's.

He calls Roselea Galilea by her nickname: "Gali cried big tears and kissed me on the cheek. She really didn't know what was going on around her. But she kissed me and she said, 'I love you,' and that's the last thing I remember."

Like Ernesto and Sandra, I faced bumps on the journey to my gurney.

The time came when I could wait no longer. My health was in the danger zone.

I had to make my final decision. I could not keep dealing with the what-ifs.

It was soon after that pushy nephrologist confronted me at the Blue Bonnet at the end of April. My transplant in Turkey was scheduled for May 16. Cindy was pushing hard for that solution, assuming that that would be the way we would go. But I was still not totally comfortable with it. I usually am not the type to feel sorry for myself, but I was facing my mortality and there was my wife, more concerned about our children than me.

Now, don't get me wrong, I would die to protect my kids.

"Yes," Cindy would say, "but you're ultimately going to subject Gregg to that very risk if you take his kidney."

So the debate between us continued to rage on the outside. And on the inside, it raged between me and myself. One of the things that really concerned me was whether having only one kidney would limit Gregg's life. He was such a fine athlete. How could I do that to him? I understood Cindy's position. Often I took it myself.

One night during those last 3 weeks, Cindy and I went out to dinner with our friends Mike Shanahan, the head coach of the Denver Broncos football team, and his wife, Peggy. Mike showed us the scar from when he had lost a kidney after getting hit too hard playing football many years before. "See," he said, pointing to the scar, "I've lived with one most of my life."

Still, Cindy wasn't able to cope with the whole idea. She simply couldn't face the reality that something had to be done. These tensions—these conflicting values, needs, and impulses—are not uncommon in transplant situations. They touch all communities.

Our rabbi, Steven Foster, offered to meet with us to help sort through these problems. By then, however, Cindy had lost her sense of spirituality. And her faith in the health care system had been shaken by her mother's death from cancer. Her lack of faith in religion and lack of faith in hospitals combined to support her preferred solution: Go to Turkey and buy that damned kidney, already!

May 16 was just around the corner. Everyone weighed in for the final round.

Dr. Kam, my surgeon at the University of Colorado Health Sciences Center, who was born in Israel, repeated his strong opposition to Dr. Shapira's Turkish alternative. "He's too old to do the surgery himself," argued Dr. Kam, "and you don't know—you have no guarantee—where his kidney actually comes from or who will actually perform the surgery."

He was not the only one working to stop my trip to Turkey. Herb Cook, my father-in-law, called everyone he could think of, again and again and again. Finally, someone at the hospital called him back. When he got off the phone, he was really excited. He reported that we could back off both the trip to Turkey and the donation of Gregg's kidney! Why? Because, he said, the woman from the hospital had told him that I was moving up on the list, after all—and indeed I would be next! I immediately called the lady Herb had spoken with, and she said he must have misunderstood. What she claimed she said to Herb was very different indeed: If a match came in and no one was ahead of me on the list, then I would get the kidney.

In other words, it was just a false alarm. A red herring. I was very disappointed, of course, but not surprised. I was simply hearing the same thing over and over again. It was just more chaos at a time when, alone on my island, I had to finally come to a decision.

People—friends and family, a doctor from Harvard, and a doctor from UCLA—were calling around the clock. One of those doctors challenged my entire approach to the problem. Why, he asked, wasn't I on dialysis? I could, he said, simply have a shunt put into my arm or chest and have a dialysis machine at home so I could simply plug myself in and do my dialysis on my own, according to my own schedule, and in perfect privacy.

Imagine, I thought, *Cindy dealing with that!* Imagine *me* dealing with that. Dialysis remained, for me, an abhorrent idea—staying still for such long periods of time, suffering the treatment's serious side effects over time, risking my ability to accept a healthy kidney down the road—I just could not accept it. And I have, in fact, been criticized by some for not taking that route while I was on the waiting list. All I can say is that it's a very personal and difficult decision.

Finally, Dr. Kam phoned me. He had gotten a call from someone at the University of Colorado who asked him why he was holding up my transplant and creating obstacles, when of course he was doing nothing of the kind. "Who said I wouldn't do it?" he asked me. "You know I'll do it anytime. I have surgery scheduled in Israel on the 18th"—2 days after I was scheduled in Turkey—"and I'll do it before I leave. Just give me the word."

That phone call with Dr. Kam, which took place in late April, pretty much made up my mind. Two days later, I called him back and we talked again, for a very long time. At the end of our call, we set a date for my surgery: May 11, only a couple of days before I was set to leave for Turkey.

At the time, I told no one that I had actually set a date with Dr. Kam to have the transplant surgery. Instead, I called Gregg and asked to meet with him. We met at the New York Deli News, down on Hampden Avenue. I asked him, "You still there for me?"

"Absolutely," he answered without hesitation, "I always knew I'd be the one."

I was more uncomfortable than ever with the idea of going to Turkey to buy that supposedly Israeli kidney. And Gregg had never been comfortable with that idea, either.

"I've got no other choice," I said. And so Gregg reaffirmed both his commitment to me and his wife Sara's support for our mutual decision.

Only then did I tell him we already had a date with the surgeon. He said it was fine. He never once complained, never reconsidered, never backed off. People ask me whether Gregg's gift to me has changed the way I feel about him. Of course I feel close to all three of my sons. I've got strong bonds with all of them.

But yes, Gregg's gift to me has made a difference in our relationship. It's not in terms of caring or closeness. It's more a matter of respect for him. And gratitude for all of his courage and support.

What many people don't know is this: Gregg actually gave me two gifts of life during that middle week of May 2004. There was the kidney he gave me, of course. But later we learned that the grandchild he would give me 9 months after our surgery was in fact conceived on the night before he went to the hospital to give me his kidney.

A deeper love I could never receive.

We talked to my other sons, Brent and Brad, and they flew in from New York near the end of April so we could have a family meeting. We had it at our home, over a dinner that no one ate. Gregg and I informed the others that we had made our decision.

Cindy insisted, "I'm not happy with this." She remained unconvinced, and remains unconvinced to this day, that we were doing the best thing. I suppose it's because she's a very stubborn person, especially when it comes to her sons. There was not much further discussion, however, after that dinner. There was, nevertheless, a lot of guilt heaped upon me, most of it by myself and Cindy. Fortunately, I did not have time to wallow in it.

Two days before the surgery, Gregg went to the hospital for more tests. Then, the day before the surgery, we went together to the hospital for our final tests. Cindy and Sara came with us. The hospital drew blood from Gregg and from me and tested the samples to see how well they would mix. Fortunately, the bloods mixed well, as was expected, given our perfect six-antigen match.

The mood was matter-of-fact. Cindy knew the decision was made and she could no longer fight it. I'm not sure who said what to whom first, but she or I or someone else must have said something to someone and word got out. A local rabbi was at the hospital making his rounds and he saw us there. He waited until the tests were over and then took Gregg and me to the hospital chapel. There we laid tefillin and prayed.

Tefillin, or phylacteries, are two small leather boxes that are worn during morning prayers by Orthodox and Conservative adult Jewish males. Each box contains parchment strips with four verses from the Torah, the Five Books of Moses. Each is attached to leather strips that are used to fasten it to the forehead or the left arm. The leather strips are wrapped around the head and arm in very precise ways. Tefillin are meant to remind the wearer of the constant presence of God and the need to always keep him uppermost in your thoughts and your deeds. Putting them on—"laying tefillin"—is both routine for those who attend morning prayers and profoundly meaningful.

Gregg had never laid tefillin before. And I hadn't done it for years, since Cindy's mom had died. There were only the three of us there in the chapel at the hospital, praying, seeking our spiritual moment. Frankly, since it was his first time—and it is a rather arcane ritual—Gregg looked a little scared to be facing medical and spiritual challenges for the first time. I think he was mainly just going through the motions for me.

After we prayed with Rabbi Cohen, we went home. I do not remember much about that last night before the transplant. But now I smile when I think of it. My first grandchild—a girl named Andie—was conceived in those hours! Gregg was having a much better time than I was.

At 5:00 in the morning I got out of bed. We had to be at the hospital by 7:00. Gregg came to the house and we went together. The mood in the car was quiet. We were apprehensive. A woman named Sarah Sewal met us at the hospital. She was the contact person sent by the hospital's Executive Program for VIPs. Sarah took us to get prepped and later stayed with my family and friends to act as an interface between them and the hospital team. In hindsight, I compare the VIP treatment we were given with the treatment received by Ernesto, Sandra, and their family. I know they got excellent medical care—but did they get the same level of hospital support that I got?

By then Cindy and Sara and a group of relatives and friends were gathering in the halls and waiting rooms. There must have been 30 of them. Who knows? There may have been more. My partner, Norm, was there with his wife, Sunny. Lynne Sullivan was there, of course. Cindy's sister Debbie and her husband, Jimmy Lustig, were there.

Just about everyone close to me was there—and then some. Frankly, the group was too big for the occasion. I couldn't see all of them, anyway.

Gregg and I were getting prepped nearby, side by side. An old friend of Gregg's, a young doctor named Mitch Robinson—whose father has been a friend of mine since college—saw Gregg from across the room. He came over to see us. He said what a "great job" Gregg was doing. It brought him to tears, and that nearly brought Gregg and me to tears.

Then surgical nurses in green scrubs wheeled us out, Gregg first, then me. I recall seeing Cindy and her sister Debbie in the hallway. And both of them were fainting, literally fainting—from nervousness, I suppose—as they wheeled us by! Debbie fell—*bang!*—right on the floor.

Only after the surgery did I learn that Debbie's head had split open. She was getting stitches in the emergency room while Gregg was giving me his kidney in the operating room.

The last thing I remember was lying down on the table.

Lynne Sullivan likes to point out that I had no idea what was really going on that morning. I was on "happy drugs," she says. She likes to tell her own version of the events, with her own buildup to the punch line.

"Let me tell you about that day," says Lynne, meaning the day of the transplant. "I saw as much of it as anyone else. Brad and Brent, Steven's other two boys, met me at the Starbucks at Third and Clayton. We were the first ones there when it opened. We got some coffee and drove to University Hospital. A woman named Sarah Sewal from the hospital's Executive Program met us there. We used to call her 'Hospital Sarah' to distinguish her from Gregg's wife, Sara. Well, Hospital Sarah took Brent, Brad, Cindy, and me away from the foyer and down to the prep area. We went into this room. It was a large room. It was the waiting room off the prep area. There were groupings of families in it. We joined Herb Cook, Cindy's father, and Jimmy Lustig, Cindy's brother-in-law, in the waiting room. Down this teeny, narrow hallway was the pre-op area."

Lynne recalls, "I saw Ernesto and his family off to one side. I had met him a few times at Jim's office, when he was still doing a lot of landscape work for Jim's company. They were so calm and happy. They were in America and Ernesto was giving the gift of life to Sandra. Cindy, in contrast, was moaning, crying—hysterical. She was holding her purse close to her chest, rocking back and forth. Her hands were cold and she had no color. She looked like she was in shock. She kept saying things like 'I just don't want this to happen.' Or, 'Why is this happening?' Or, 'Why does my son have to do this? I can't go through this. I'm so mad at Steven for putting my son through this.' It was all simply beyond her comprehension. I thought she would throw up or faint. So I asked her, 'When was the last time you ate?' I could see her blood sugar was out of whack. I made her take a bite or two of an Atkins bar. And she had some Diet Coke. But this went on for a long time—45 minutes at least. Finally, they said the family could go back to see Steven and Gregg in the prep area before they wheeled them out."

Lynne says, "I told Cindy before she went back there, 'You be strong. Don't let Gregg see you cry. Give Steven a hug and a kiss and tell him you love him. Be strong.' Then Cindy and Brent and Brad went down the tiny, narrow hallway to the prep area to say good-bye to Steven and Gregg before they were taken off to surgery."

The hallway was tiny enough and the waiting room was close enough that Lynne could see past the open curtain that barely separated the prep area from the hallway. She could see that Cindy was getting hysterical again so she guided Cindy away from us and back into the hallway.

Today, Lynne laughs about it. "You know, when Steven tells the story, he gets a couple of the details wrong. You have to understand that he was flat on his back watching Gregg get wheeled out first. His field of vision was very limited. All he really saw was the top of Gregg's head going down that little hallway. Besides, he was on happy drugs and by then he didn't know what was happening. So, first off, Debbie Lustig wasn't even there yet. She didn't faint and hit her head at the hospital. I know because I saw Debbie when she arrived some time later. She got off the elevator, after we'd been taken to a different waiting room upstairs, wearing some sort of fancy Escada outfit with blood matted in her hair. She must have fallen down at home or somewhere else. I don't know. But I do know she wasn't there when they wheeled Gregg out. Though Steven is right, Debbie was getting her head stitched up in the emergency room while he was getting a kidney from Gregg."

At this point Lynne smiles a big smile. "And Cindy never fainted when they wheeled Gregg out of the prep area and into the hallway. Here's what really happened. Jimmy Lustig and Herb Cook and Rick and Shelley Sapkin"—Cindy and Debbie's other sister and brother-in-law—"were all there, of course. Cindy had so much adrenaline going though her, she was ready to lunge onto that gurney with her son on it. She was literally going to throw herself on him. So I tackled her from behind. I did. I jumped at her from behind and wrapped my arms around her and pulled her away from the gurney. We fell backwards and down, though we never actually hit the floor. From Steven's vantage point it might have looked like Cindy had fainted. Or fallen out of the picture. Or someone told him the story wrong. Either way, that is how it really happened. I can remember Cindy felt so strong when she was trying to pull herself away from me. And I just kept saying to her, 'Be strong. Tell him you love him.' It was a huge drama."

Ernesto's family saw it all. And throughout they remained quiet and reserved. "They were more spiritual," says Lynne, "and more religious. They were thrilled with the gift of life. They were thanking their God. They just could not understand all the hand-wringing. Science and medicine were bringing their loved one a chance to live. Didn't those people—meaning us—understand that?"

Next, according to Lynne, I was wheeled out of the prep area, into the hallway, and off to the operating theater. The family settled down and Hospital Sarah led them to another waiting room on the fourth floor, next to the recovery and intensive care areas. Ernesto's family had not yet been brought up because his and Sandra's surgeries would come after Gregg's and mine. But there was a woman and her young daughter waiting for her husband, who was having a liver transplant.

Soon it was clear: The drama was far from over. Family and friends were pacing. Everyone was nervous. Cindy was in shock. Off to the side, Hospital Sarah would get updates from the operating theater and explain to Lynne and others who would listen, "Now this is what is happening. Steve is out cold. Gregg's kidney has been removed. They're getting ready to make the switch." It was a running commentary.

Finally, the surgeries were done. Everything had gone well. Lynne says, "I felt like 100 pounds of bricks had been lifted from my shoulders. All that weight was gone. I felt relaxed for the first time in hours, days—even weeks."

And then the circus came to town. It wasn't enough that my entourage of 30 was already encamped at the hospital to support me. Now, with the transplant done, everyone in Denver who had been told not to come to the hospital showed up. There were friends of friends, business acquaintances, all sorts of people who were not part of my inner circle and really had no business coming on the very day of the surgery.

"It was a drama-fest," laughs Lynne. "There was enough food to feed a small country. The delivery guy from Pasta Pasta Pasta somehow got hurt in the elevator and was down in the emergency room getting patched up while Steven was getting his kidney and Debbie was getting her stitches."

So Lynne spent her time text messaging and talking to Jim, her husband, who claimed he would have liked to have been there, but couldn't stand to witness the show. My partner, Norm Brownstein, was working the phones, calling clients and friends to report on my progress. "And Cindy had all her girlfriends around her," says Lynne. "Really, it got totally out of control and turned into this big, loud, disgusting party. Gregg's wife, Sara, and the friend she had with her were a bit taken aback, I think."

It's easy to wonder how Lynne avoids the stereotypes of the people who cling to her friends like magnets. She does, after all, sport her own share of diamonds, and none could be called particularly modest. She used to fly in Jim's private plane, owned by a company Carolyn cooked up and called Gorilla Aviation. It's not a modest lifestyle.

Then you notice the simple plastic bracelet she wears on her wrist. It's one of those ubiquitous bracelets in support of this cause or that. But this one is not Lance Armstrong yellow. Lynne's bracelet is bright green. It says *"Done Vida"* in Latin and "Donate Life" in English. It's for donors of blood, tissue, or organs, or those who commit to be donors. Lynne wears her bracelet as naturally as her dark hair and her diamonds.

"My most poignant experience," she says, "my own drama among all the dramas, was a much quieter moment. It was much later in the day. Steven and Gregg had come back from surgery. They were in their rooms. Hospital Sarah had let Cindy and Sara go in to see them for a few minutes, then she said everyone had to leave. We took Cindy home and tried to get her to lie down. Finally she slept for a couple of hours. Then she got up and we all went back to the hospital. They let us look in on Steven and Gregg. One by one, so I did it alone. Gregg looked just fine. He was sound asleep."

And here Lynne pauses to wipe the tears welling in her eyes. More accurately, she pats them down, perhaps to conserve their moisture. "Then I looked in on Steven."

Lynne's face crumples. She sobs openly as she remembers, "His face was pink. He looked so good, so immediately. The transplant—it had taken! It was instantaneous! I had seen him the night before and he had been so weak, so jaundiced, so yellow. Now, there he was, looking so healthy, so quickly. It was so incredible. I thought, *To be able with our science to create this chance for life!* I was overwhelmed. It was so amazing."

When Sandra woke up after her transplant, she was glad it was over. She was grateful to Ernesto and happy to be alive. She had some pain around the incision, but her recovery went well, both in the days after the surgery and over the next months. During her stay at University Hospital, she did not have an entourage to entertain or a hallway full of visitors. Just her immediate family. She has always been a very private person. She never wanted other people to know what was happening to her and hadn't told her friends about her kidney transplant before it happened.

CHAPTER TEN

FATALLY FLAWED

The first thing I remember when I woke up was Cindy standing next to my bed, staring down at me, looking frustrated and concerned. She said, "Gregg is miserable. He's in terrible pain. See what you did to him?"

Somehow I knew she was overreacting out of love and concern for our son. Still, there I was, coming out of my anesthetic stupor, feeling pretty damn miserable myself and hearing this!

All I could muster in response was, "What do you want me to do about it now?"

The exchange between Cindy and me was symbolic. The transplant may have solved my immediate medical problem, but now other needs were clamoring for attention. I was alive and my prognosis was good. And everyone wanted a piece of the action.

The attention was overwhelming. I woke up in a floral shop. There were so many flowers that it was hard for the doctors and nurses to move freely around the room. The sweet floral scents overpowered the hospital's harsh antiseptic smells. Cindy and Lynne ended up sending a lot of those flowers down the hall to Ernesto and Sandra, whose surgeries had gone routinely and whose recoveries would go quickly.

Indeed, the line between people thinking they were being helpful and concerned and people becoming intrusive sometimes got pretty thin. So many people came to visit. Some of them I had not seen for 5 or 6 years. Some were truly close friends of ours, and some were truly no more than acquaintances. The local newspapers all ran stories.

But it was hard to be social. At first I was in pain, and the pain and the drugs made me slip in and out of consciousness. Sometimes I would wake up and there would be people in the room and I knew I could not deal with them, so I faked being asleep.

By the 2nd day after the surgery, I was getting out of bed and walking around. The doctors were encouraging me to start some limited activity. I was hoping I could go home in the normal range of 3 to 5 days. Then an odd incident made it 10.

On the 3rd day after the surgery, I awoke early in the morning. The light in the room was dim. But I could tell no one else was in the room—except for a lone woman. She was standing over my bed, looking down at me. But it was not Cindy. And it was not any of the medical staff.

It was the wife of a friend! I had no idea why this woman would be in my room at that early hour, all alone. I still have no idea. Suddenly a nurse appeared and asked, "Are you okay?"

"Yeah," I answered, "why?"

By then my visitor had disappeared or been taken away.

The nurse persisted, "You don't feel any different?"

"Well, yeah," I repeated, "why?"

"Because you're in fibrillation," she said. She had been monitoring my heart from her station in the hallway, and when I woke up and saw my friend's wife standing over me, my heart must have started racing or twitching. As a result, my doctors kept me in the hospital for an extra week to make sure it didn't happen again, and I was none too happy about it.

Still, my recovery went well. Three days after the surgery, the pain was subsiding for both me and Gregg. Cindy, in fact, had been right. Gregg had experienced quite a lot of pain for the first couple of days. Even his wife, Sara, had been upset because he was in so much pain at first. But within 2 weeks he was playing ball again, and he suffered absolutely no complications. Fortunately, neither did I.

After a few days I was taking laps through the hospital halls. I had lost 12 or 13 pounds and soon I began recovering my weight—or 10 pounds of it—slowly.

I was put on prednisone, a corticosteroid similar to a natural hormone produced by the adrenal gland. It is widely used for many purposes, but it has many side effects. That swollen, "moon face" look of Jerry Lewis's comes from prednisone. Other side effects include stomach irritation, vomiting, headaches, dizziness, insomnia, depression, acne, increased hair growth, muscle weakness, colds, and infections that last a long time.

Think about the last two. Colds and infections last a long time because prednisone is used, in organ transplant cases, to suppress the recipient's immune system. It lessens the chances of organ rejection. But, to avoid those nasty side effects, the less you take, the better. I went from 20 milligrams a day to 5 milligrams soon after the transplant. Since Gregg was such a good match for me, I never had a great risk of rejecting his kidney.

Still, those side effects were very real. After 2 or 3 months, prednisone can start adversely affecting your organs. It gave me cholesterol problems and increased my blood sugar. It made me into a type 2 diabetic, which I had been warned about. At first my doctors wanted me to test my blood and give myself insulin injections before every meal, but I have never followed their orders that strictly—and I have never done it more than once a day. I still do it every morning, though I believe a healthy diet and active lifestyle are as important as the insulin in controlling my diabetes.

For the first couple of weeks after I left the hospital, I still felt sore and swollen. I'd have to learn to manage the long-term effects of the transplant, but the 7-inch scar across my groin, the nerves they had to cut in my leg, and all of the drugs and their strange side effects were well worth it. I was alive! And had a new, healthy kidney!

I started walking to build myself back up. I had to get strong so my body could fight off infections while its immune system was being suppressed. At first, I went only a quarter of a mile each day. Then half a mile, then more. By 5 weeks after the surgery, I was able to attend a friend's wedding and dance one dance. In July, about 8 weeks after the transplant, I started working out with light weights and a stationary bike at home. I could go out to the movies, too. But there was a "but," and it was a big one.

Because I was susceptible to infections, my doctors said I should avoid crowds and touching. But shaking hands—schmoozing—is my whole life. I find myself in a lot of crowds and can't avoid shaking hands. So, to this day, I have to wash my hands constantly to avoid infection.

I started going back to the office after 3 weeks. At first it was for just a couple of hours a week, but then I built up to 6 hours a day for a month, and 9 months later I was back to 10 to 12 hours of being on duty each day.

During this time I got to be friends with my two doctors, nephrologist Larry Chan, MD, and surgeon Igal Kam, MD. Larry is an active Democrat, so when Bill Clinton called to ask me to host that fund-raiser for the Clinton Library, I invited both him and Igal.

The fund-raiser was held at my home on July 12, 2 months after the transplant. President Clinton was in Denver to give a reading from his new autobiography at the Tattered Cover Bookstore later that day. I hosted 50 people for a lunch, including former Denver mayor Wellington Webb and his wife, Wilma; Ken Salazar, who in November would be elected Colorado's newest US senator and is now President Barack Obama's secretary of the interior; current Denver mayor John Hickenlooper; and Mary Ricketson, dean of the

University of Denver College of Law. Together, we raised $400,000 for the Clinton Library during that lunch.

I was starting to feel better, and Cindy was being more support-ive during my recovery than she had been before. In August I started playing golf again. I went to the Cherry Creek Country Club and golfed nine holes. I let myself use the women's tee and shot a 38, which I thought was pretty good.

I also started to reenter public life. The media were calling a lot. Penny Parker from the *Rocky Mountain News* and Bill Husted from the *Denver Post* had been covering my surgery and my recovery. I even chaired a big Children's Hospital dinner in September. It was a daunt-ing obligation, but I had agreed to it the year before and could not say no. Fortunately, my staff worked hard to help me out. Our entertain-ment was Donna Summers, and it became the most successful dinner in the hospital's history. We raised $1.6 million in one night!

In October, my friend Don Kortz, the past chairman of the board of the Denver Chamber of Commerce, called me to say, "The Cham-ber is going to give Norm"—meaning Norm Brownstein, my part-ner and close friend—"an award at this year's annual awards luncheon. You have to make sure he comes."

I agreed. I told Don I would go with Norm to the luncheon to make sure he would show up. When the date arrived, I walked with him from our office building to the nearby hotel where the event was being held. As we entered the hotel lobby, an odd thing hap-pened. A woman named Molly, who runs a high-end women's cloth-ing store downtown, came up to me and said, "Oh, Steve, I just saw your wife."

I figured she must have mistaken Norm's wife, Sunny, for my wife, Cindy. Both are blonde and of similar build. Both are seen often in public. It was a common mistake.

Then someone else approached and said, "Congratulations, Steve," but I figured all he was saying was the sort of congratulations you receive when someone close to you achieves something great—like something said at your kid's graduation or wedding.

Finally, at the end of the presentations, Kirk McDonald from the Denver Newspaper Agency was called to the podium to accept the award I had thought Norm was supposed to receive. I turned to Norm and said, "I have to confess. I'm not sure how it's going down, but it was my job to get you here today so you could accept an award."

Norm—big guy, big presence—smiled one of his coy little smiles and said, "No, Steve, I'm the one who has to confess. You're here because of an award, all right, but I'm not the one who's getting it. You're the one who's getting it. You're this year's recipient of the Del Hock award for a lifetime of public service!"

I was shocked. I did not know. In fact, all along it had been Norm's job to make sure I showed up at the lunch, and he had contrived to get me there under false pretenses.

My whole family was there, of course—Cindy and my three sons. They showed a short film about me and my life. Then a speaker talked about his "five heroes."

And when I went up to the podium to accept the award, I made it clear that I, too, had a hero. I said into the microphone, "My hero is my son Gregg."

Gregg gave me his kidney and the gift of life. And when you receive an award for "lifetime achievement," you can't help but think, *Wait a minute, is this supposed to be the end of it all?* I say no! And my denial has nothing to do with a fear of death.

I've always believed in reincarnation or a better life after death, even though those aren't really Jewish concepts. My life has included so many episodes of coincidence and déjà vu that I can't help but think there's a string or a thread—or a purpose, as my mother called it—that keeps things connected and ties things together. That drives life along.

When you are a public figure living outside the mainstream and you face your mortality like I did, you come away feeling blessed. You ask yourself how you want to spend the next 5 or 10 years of your life. You begin to broaden your perspectives. You think more and more about the choices other people have to face.

For example, because kidney disease knows no demographic boundaries, I have had the opportunity to meet a lot of different people from different walks of life by just going to my doctor's office to get my blood tested. At first after the transplant, I had to go 5 days a week. After 3 weeks, I had to go three times a week. Then it went down to twice a week, then once a week. Finally, it was once a month.

While sitting in the waiting room, I got to know some of the other regulars. There was this African American guy who always used to laugh and say he was related to a Latino guy "through our organs." And there was another middle-aged man whose recovery had not gone very well. He had to take a lot more immunosuppressant drugs than me, and they were keeping him weak. He said he had not worked in the 2 years since his kidney transplant.

When I told this man that I had gone back to work after only a few weeks, all he could do was look down sadly and say, "Geez."

Sometimes I get distressed by the willingness of some patients to allow their transplants to limit them so in their activities. I have found that some of these people use their transplants as an excuse not to work, not to play, and not to get on with their lives. Of course, I was a lot luckier than many of them. I had gotten a perfectly matched organ from a healthy live donor. I was better able than most to get on with my life as it had been before my transplant.

That autumn, things were going very well. I was feeling great. One Saturday morning, I played tennis with my regular tennis partner, David Engleberg. It was chilly that day, so we played indoors at

Racquet World at Yale and Monaco. I had been easing back into my physical activities and was proud to be able to play for 2 whole hours.

I drove home and told Brent, who was in town from New York, that I was going to clean up and after that we could go to Deli Tech for some lunch. I had worked up quite an appetite. I went into the bathroom, closed the door, stood over the toilet bowl, and peed. A bright red flow of blood was all that came out. My heart stopped.

The water in the toilet turned pink, then red. There was no pain. But there was a crushing fear. Not fear for my life—fear, rather, that I was rejecting Gregg's kidney.

I stood there thinking, *First I take his kidney, now it doesn't work! I've wasted his organ!* I was totally concerned for Gregg, not myself. I was heaping blame upon myself. Then I realized that I had to stay calm. I knew I could not go out there and tell Brent what was going on. Or what I was fearing. He would freak out. I had to disguise my alarm.

I finished cleaning up, composed myself, and went out to face Brent. I said as casually as I could, "You know, on second thought, I think I have to pass on lunch."

"Why?" he asked. I could tell his antennae were up.

"Oh," I said as casually as I could, "I just think I should go to the hospital and have something checked."

Now Brent's antennae were twitching. "What's wrong?" he asked, concerned.

"Just some blood in my urine," I said. I didn't tell him about the stream of bright red blood that had arched into the toilet, or about the fear I was feeling inside.

"I'll go with you, Dad," he said.

"No, no," I insisted. "I'm okay. Really. I'll just drive myself."

Behind the steering wheel, I was actually thankful to be away from my home and my family so I could face my fear without having to worry about their reactions. I took a long, deep breath and called Dr. Chan on my cell phone.

He answered. I told him what had happened. "How do you feel?" he asked.

"Fine," I answered. "Maybe a little tired. I've been playing tennis. We did 2 hours this morning."

"And was it pink or red?" he asked. We both knew it was not unusual to have a little blood in your urine after a kidney transplant. I had already had some. Enough to turn the water pink, but not enough to turn it . . .

"Red," I said. "Bright red."

"Okay," said Dr. Chan, "come to the hospital. I'll meet you there."

Soon I got to the emergency room. They did a urinalysis. And it was still bright red. So they put me on a glucose and water drip—a very fast drip. They meant to put a gallon of fluids into me quickly to flush out whatever was there.

Meanwhile, they also did an ultrasound, but they saw nothing alarming. Just my two old nonfunctioning kidneys and my new functioning one. That's right. Usually your kidneys are not taken out when you have a transplant. They just move them over and tuck the new one into place. Over time, the old ones shrink.

Dr. Chan remained calm. I remained alarmed. "It could be the Coumadin," he speculated. That was the blood thinner I was taking as part of the carefully concocted cocktail of chemicals Dr. Chan had prescribed for me after the transplant. I was taking about 15 pills each day at that time: prednisone, Myfortic, and Rapamune to suppress my immune system; metoprolol, Lanoxin, and Coumadin to thin my blood and control my heart rhythm; Lipitor and Pravachol to control my cholesterol—and who knows what else! Today, I take a lot fewer pills, but at the time I was still full of drugs.

Dr. Chan had explained all about each of them. When it came to the Coumadin, he said that I had to be careful not to cut myself. With blood thinners in my system, I could bleed for hours if I did. I should even avoid using a straightedge razor when I shaved, he said, though I continued to use one, despite his warning. Now he was speculating that the blood in my urine could have been caused by the Coumadin.

"Or a blood clot," he said.

"Blood clot?"

"Yes," he said. "Your body always has blood clots in it from former injuries, from . . . whatever. It's all very natural. Especially after surgery. So the Coumadin could have loosened or released a blood clot somewhere. Or it could've happened on its own."

We never knew what caused the alarm. But after 2 very nervous hours of glucose and water dripping fast into my veins, the color of my urine began to turn lighter. We saw it go from bright red to red, then from dark pink to pink. And finally, thankfully, to clear. The emergency was past. I breathed a deep sigh of relief.

Laurence Chan, MD, is the director of transplant nephrology at the University of Colorado Health Sciences Center. He works closely with Dr. Kam. The man from Israel wields the knife and the man from Hong Kong prescribes the drugs. Of course, it's a bit more complex than that.

It is actually quite an art, mixing the drugs for kidney transplant patients. The cocktail must be carefully tailored to each patient's needs. For example, I was able to take fewer immunosuppressant drugs than many because I received a perfectly matched kidney from my son. The drugs must also be monitored. If too many are prescribed or their dosages are too strong, they can damage the new organ and the transplant goes for naught.

Dr. Chan is the man who does the tailoring and monitoring. He's the doctor who the patient sees before, during, and after the surgery. He also chairs his hospital's donor selection committee, which means he's the guy who applies all the fancy formulas and objective criteria to specific cases. When elements of subjectivity creep into the process, as they often do, that subjectivity is guided by Larry Chan's wealth of experience.

He is a font of knowledge. He has to be, in order to prevent complications, prescribe the right cocktail of drugs, and perform his medical mission. Ask him how many people need kidney transplants in America and he will tell you it's many more than the 70,000-plus on the waiting list. He will remind you that not everyone qualifies to be on the waiting list. He will tell you that there are more than 500,000 people on dialysis and that they would enjoy a far better quality of life with a transplant.

Dr. Chan can describe the development of immunosuppressant drugs, from early corticosteroids to cyclosporine in the 1980s, to tacrolimus and mycophenolate in the 1990s, to Myfortic and rapamycin in the 2000s. In his technical presentations, he refers to transplants as "grafts"—the same term that appeared repeatedly in the Web site for the notorious "transplant outlaw" Dr. Zaki Shapira.

According to Dr. Chan, organ transplants actually grew out of innovations in skin grafting developed during World War II for treating burn victims. He seems to know everything. He has been in the transplant business for more than 30 years and has seen it all. And, like many who have seen it all, the man delivering the information is often more interesting than the information itself. Born in 1947 to ethnic Chinese parents, he decided to remain in Hong Kong after his family moved to California in the 1960s. He visited them there, he explains, but he just couldn't "get into the scene."

After earning his medical degree at the University of Hong Kong, Dr. Chan headed to England for his residency at the University of Edinburgh and a fellowship at Oxford, where he studied with transplant pioneers Sir Roy Calne and Sir Peter Morris. He received another fellowship in 1982 that brought him to America and Harvard's Peter Bent Brigham Hospital in Boston.

Dr. Chan works with the Transplantation Society, an international association that pursues a wide range of issues ranging from the medical—minimizing complications, developing new drugs, enhancing quality of life—to the ethical—who should finance organ transplants, for example, and how we can expand and optimize the donor pool.[1] Still, for all of his knowledge and experience, what matters the most to Dr. Chan is the caring, "the worrying about patients," he says.

To illustrate, he recalls a case from the early 1980s, when there were fewer drugs available to aid the transplant process, so the mixing of the medications was especially critical. And making the drugs available to the patient so they could be taken in the proper sequence was equally critical.

It was Thanksgiving. A kidney recipient named José Avila lived in Alamosa, several hours south of Denver in the San Luis Valley. José had to drive back and forth from Alamosa to Denver to get his medications. But the weather was getting bad and he couldn't make it all the way. Now, Dr. Chan had gotten to know José pretty well by then. Providing psychological support came with the job. And it made Dr. Chan feel good to know that patients like José could look to him for that support. So when José called with his problem, Dr. Chan got into his big Toyota Land Cruiser and drove for 3 hours to meet José halfway in Pueblo and deliver his drugs personally. They met at a small truck stop outside the city and shared a hot cup of coffee in its coffee shop.

José was in his early thirties. He had a small build and a "sleeping" kidney, which meant that his kidney transplant appeared to have taken, but the kidney was slow in getting started. It had decreased functioning, so the drugs were all the more important to prevent rejection. José did just fine.

Then there were the cases that combined the personal rewards with the professional challenges. Later in the 1980s, Dr. Chan faced one of these cases. He had a patient whose transplanted kidney wasn't working well. Finally, it failed. The patient needed another transplant. But Dr. Chan felt it was important to know why the transplanted kidney had failed. What was the cause of the failure? Unless he could figure that out, another transplant could be nothing more than a waste of another good organ.

And Dr. Chan liked nothing more than to make a challenging diagnosis correctly.

He suspected the answer was oxalosis, the result of a rare metabolic disease that had not been previously diagnosed in the patient or his family. A genetic defect causes a deficiency of an enzyme in the liver, which eventually leads to kidney failure and a buildup of oxalate in the blood. To demonstrate that his diagnosis was correct, Dr. Chan developed his own method of measuring oxalate. In doing this he drew on his long-standing interest in chemistry.

"I started out as a chemistry machine," he says. "I studied biochemistry. It was my research interest. I focused on the nature of cell injury—injury on a cellular level. Later, I merged my interest in chemistry with my interest in transplantation. I helped design a better chemical preservation fluid to stop the donated kidney from going sour."

So, with his new method of measuring oxalate, Dr. Chan could explain to his patient and his colleagues why the first kidney transplant had gone bad. It was because the patient also needed a liver transplant. That made the case even more challenging.

Dr. Chan became the patient's cheerleader, urging patience, telling him the organs would come. And they did. Another surgery was performed, this time transplanting both a kidney and a liver into the patient. Dr. Chan recalls that the guy was a Vietnam vet who wanted so much to lead an active, normal life. The second round of transplants worked perfectly. In April 2005 Dr. Chan saw this patient, then in his seventies, and the man was still doing great. It was another personal and professional victory.

And as for me, Dr. Chan—a thin man with a twinkle in his eyes—says, "Steve is such a wonderful patient. He listens and remembers. And such discipline!"

Like Dr. Kam, Dr. Chan opposed my going to Turkey to buy that supposedly Israeli kidney from Dr. Zaki Shapira. "With so much risk and uncertainty," he explains, "I told Steve we should do whatever we could do here first. There was still time."

Yet Dr. Chan is a realist. He sees the pressures encouraging markets in organs. He sees the relationship between those markets and the Internet. He knows the pendulum is swinging, but he thinks that commercialization of organs is bad for several reasons. The first is the safety factor. There are simply no controls to keep diseased organs out of the marketplace. Then, of course, there are the cultural and religious problems.

Instead of commercialization, Dr. Chan sees a different future. He looks forward to innovations in utilizing the organs of older deceased donors. He foresees a time when we not only accept "kidney swaps," but also nonpaired or delayed exchanges. He also predicts advances in transplants using organs that do not have good cross-matching of blood type. "Why not take the risk?" he asks. With all the new drugs available to condition the body before surgery, new plasma exchange techniques, and new types of therapies, the pool of available organs could be increased significantly.

Then there's stem cell research, which Dr. Chan sees as the biggest thing in the near future. "Cell transplants" will be used, he says, at first to heal brain and spinal cord injuries. Soon stem cells will be used to help organs like kidneys and livers regenerate. Already in the few years since my surgery there have been advances in this area.

"Someday," he says, his eyes sparkling, "we will have totally artificial organs." Or more accurately, he explains, we will likely merge stem cells with artificial machines. We will create new membranes—the filters that cleanse the blood—that are far more sophisticated than today's commercially available dialysis membranes. These will be called "bioreactors." We will see machine technology converge with transplant technology. "We will prevent end-stage organ failure," predicts Dr. Chan.

Yet his story about José sticks with me more than his dazzling predictions because that story reminds me of the story of Ernesto and Sandra. They, like José, occupy a different part of the social and economic structure. Their challenges are very different from mine. In the case of José, he faced the geographical disadvantages of the rural health care system and struggled to connect with Dr. Chan's more urban system. In the case of Ernesto and Sandra, they faced all the complexities of an imperfect public health care system that provided them with far less personalized attention than I got.

Still, Ernesto and Sandra never complain. They are young and robust. Ernesto was back at work and feeling great within days after his operation. And Sandra never faced the danger of a relapse. Her recovery went well. But the differences between their situation and mine haunt me. It's one of the reasons I collaborated on this book.

Fortunately, President Obama's new administration is working hard on health care reform so those differences can begin to disappear. I hope the results satisfy three conditions: First, the United States should establish a minimum level of universal health care that is available to everyone without regard to income. Do it through the insurance companies. Do it through a partial socialization of medicine. But do it. Second, the United States should encourage employers to provide group insurance–based health care in a far more effective and streamlined manner. If that means providing them with direct subsidies, what better way is there to spend tax dollars than on public health? Third, the US health care system must retain enough of its market-based capitalist roots to allow those who can afford it to seek private health care or enhanced insurance coverage at their own expense if they choose to.

In whatever way health care reform evolves in America, we should learn the lessons taught by other countries. Cuba, for instance, has a basic health care system that puts primary care providers in every neighborhood and emphasizes preventive care. That seems to me like a good place to start. But wherever we start, we must be sure to cover everyone in our nation, rich and poor. Basic health care is a human right.

Kidney disease is indiscriminate. It comes in many forms. It attacks the rich and poor alike, the famous and the unknown. It killed actress Sandra Dee. It forced fashion guru Steven Cojocaru of *Entertainment Tonight* to get two transplants.

Five months after Gregg donated his kidney to me and Ernesto donated his kidney to his sister Sandra, a very different transplant drama took place in Denver. For the first time, a kidney donor and recipient were matched by a commercial Web site.[2] Bob Hickey, 58, of Edwards, Colorado, had waited for more than 5 years for his transplant. His solution came when he was linked with Samuel Robert Smitty, 32, of Chattanooga, Tennessee. They were paired by MatchingDonors.com, a Web site created only 10 months before to match donors with patients—for a fee.

That's right. It was a *commercial* Web site that charged a fee for patients to post their profiles on it. And it dealt only with live donors. Hickey paid the Web site $295 per month for 3 months. He also paid roughly $5,000 to Smitty to cover his travel costs, lost wages, and medical costs.

But he did not pay for the organ itself. That would have been illegal.

At first, both Dr. Kam, the transplant surgeon, and Presbyterian/St. Luke's Hospital balked. The surgery was delayed for a day so the ethics could be debated. Then both doctor and hospital relented and the transplant was performed. Supporters and critics quickly weighed in. Activists defended the practice, pointing to the advent of private advertising for organs and Pennsylvania's new program to allow payments to families of deceased donors to help cover funeral expenses, as well as the increasing pressure being put on Congress to expand experimental programs designed to stimulate organ donation.[3]

Medical ethicists countered with a vengeance. While no laws actually prohibited the solicitation of live organ donations, cries of foul came from the United Network for Organ Sharing (UNOS), the organization that administers America's only Organ Procurement and Transplantation Network.[4]

"[The Web site] exploits vulnerable populations and subverts the equitable allocation of organs for transplantation," said a UNOS spokesperson at the time.

The American Society of Transplant Surgeons called upon its 1,000 members to boycott transplants arranged and performed outside widely accepted medical industry standards.[5] The critics were not interested in hearing about the hospital's reasons for granting a "compassionate exemption."[6] Yet all the while, Hickey and Smitty believed they had acted within the letter of the law.

Smitty vigorously denied that he had sold his kidney. He invited scrutiny of his finances. He said, "If [an investigator] finds out that I received one penny more than I'm allowed, I'll kiss her behind."[7] He also said he was on a "quest" to do something right since his wife's mother had died a year before.

His invitation backfired. Scrutiny revealed that Smitty had a criminal past. He once was convicted for selling LSD. He was frequently behind in his child support payments. When he returned to

Tennessee, he was promptly jailed. He went from being a national hero to a deadbeat overnight. The ethicists licked their chops.

Afterward, Dr. Kam discussed his dilemma with me. At first he had refused simply because the ethics board had not yet cleared the procedure. If he had moved forward without his ethics board's approval, he knew he risked doing something that could be unethical, maybe even illegal. For him, it was purely an internal hospital matter. Once the board gave its ruling, he went ahead and performed the transplant.

Dr. Kam is a highly skilled and well-respected surgeon. Silver-haired and stout, he looks a little like Marlon Brando circa *Last Tango in Paris*. He was born and educated in Haifa. And if Beirut is the Paris of the Middle East, then Haifa is its San Francisco, for Haifa is the most integrated of the major cities in Israel. It is built over a busy port that rises to majestic Mount Carmel. It is very big on commerce and technology.

The Technion–Israel Institute of Technology at Technion City spreads across Mount Carmel.[8] Technion is the MIT of Israel, founded decades before the country's independence. From DNA to software to Nobel laureates, Technion is the place. Its Web site boasts that of every 10,000 workers in Israel, 135 are scientists or engineers, whereas the United States ranks a distant second with only 85 out of 10,000!

Technion City houses both the technical institute and the biggest concentration of high-tech start-up companies outside Silicon Valley. In a world "flattened" by the spread of market-based economies[9] and new forms of communication, India and China may attract outsourcing due to their sheer numbers. But Israel attracts the innovators at the top of the scientific food chain. Dr. Kam is one of those innovators.[10] He earned his clinical medical degree from Technion and performed his residency at Rambam Medical Center in Haifa.

Then, he received a fellowship that brought him to America and changed his life.

In 1984, at the University of Pittsburgh, Dr. Kam got to study organ transplantation under Thomas Starzl, MD, one of the pioneers of transplant surgery. Dr. Starzl had performed the first liver transplant at the University of Colorado, and at his urging, Dr. Kam moved to Denver in 1988. He's now the chief of transplant surgery and professor of surgery at the University of Colorado Health Sciences Center. Formerly a member of the UNOS Liver and Intestinal Organ Transplantation Committee, Dr. Kam is hardly a renegade—though he has been known to ride a Harley and listen to Springsteen during surgery!

In January 2004, less than a year before his encounter with Hickey and Smitty, the *Denver Post* ran an article comparing MatchingDonors.com with LifeSharers.com, a different group that charged no fees but created a membership system in which members commit to donating their organs to other members upon their death. In the article, Dr. Kam stated, "I think it's all right if you are a donor and you want to donate and select where the kidney goes, as long as there is no financial compensation for the donor."[11] Later, after Hickey and Smitty put his ethics to the test, the *Rocky Mountain News* quoted Dr. Kam as saying, "It's a questionable way to recruit donors. . . . A dangerous way. When you're buying something on [the Internet], you never know exactly what you are getting."[12]

Today Dr. Kam explains, "If anybody really wants to donate a kidney, he can go to a kidney transplant program, knock on the door, and say, 'I'm here to donate one of my kidneys.' It's already happening here in America. We call them Good Samaritan donors. But if we open it up and let people negotiate—donors and recipients over the Internet—we create the risk that money will be exchanged for the organ itself."[13]

On December 23, 2004, 2 months after the MatchingDonors.com

controversy, the medical community celebrated the 50th anniversary of the first kidney transplant.[14] Eleven years after that historic surgery, one of Dr. Kam's mentors, Dr. Starzl, performed the first liver transplant. And by 2005, the University of Colorado Health Sciences Center had completed its 1,000th liver transplant and more than 1,500 kidney transplants.

Like his mentor, Dr. Kam gets excited about live donor liver transplants: "[They're] one of the hottest issues . . . at transplant meetings."[15] Like kidneys, livers can be transplanted from live donors. With kidneys, they take one of the donor's two organs in its entirety. With livers, they take a segment of the healthy organ and, if all goes well, the donor's liver regenerates while the transplanted segment generates a new liver in the recipient. Live donor liver transplants are difficult, however. Dr. Kam proudly notes that University Hospital was the first in the United States to use the most current technique. He says, "This is hard surgery that requires a lot of experience."

On that 50th anniversary of organ transplants, Dr. Kam said, "Transplants have almost become routine procedures. Everyone who gets a new organ, it makes them so happy. Important judges in town have received livers, big lawyers have had kidney transplants. And, of course, all the people you don't hear about."[16]

He might as well have said, "The peasant and the power broker alike."

Eight months after my transplant, I took my family to Maui for winter vacation. We have been going to Hawaii with friends from Denver for as long as I can recall—except for that one time when we went to Mexico. One day I was sitting by the swimming pool with Nancy Davis, the daughter of Marvin Davis, the Denver billionaire who died a few years ago. Marvin used to have an office in the same building as my firm. I did business with him and saw close-up his rise from oilman to owner of 20th Century Fox.

Nancy asked me to call her friend, Steven Cojocaru, the fashion and style guru often seen on television and in *People* magazine. Cojo was suffering from polycystic kidney disease and needed a transplant. He was very depressed over the prospect, and Nancy thought I could cheer him up and walk him through the process.

So I called him and, sure enough, he was depressed. He said he'd finally reached the top in his career, and now this kidney business was going to ruin it all. He told me he had a friend who was a good match and willing to be a donor, but he did not know if his friend would go through with it. I gave him a pep talk, told him how much better he'd feel after the transplant, and encouraged him to get it done so he could start his recovery. We struck up a friendship. He did go forward and received his friend's kidney.

But Cojo's recovery did not go as smoothly as mine. His friend was a good match but not a close relative, so not a perfect match. He had to take a lot more immunosuppressant drugs than I did. It lowered his resistance to infection, so his doctors said he could not have his dog around for some time. I have never heard him get as excited as when he told me the doctors had finally said his dog could come home.

Unfortunately, Cojo caught an infection that destroyed his first transplanted kidney, so his mother had to step in and donate a second organ to him. He talks all about it in his recent memoir.[17] At the time, before his first transplant, he had less weighty concerns: Would he make it to the Academy Awards show? When would he be healthy again?

I told him, "There are two keys to your recovery. One is your mind. You have to take control of your attitude. You have to be positive and stay focused on building yourself back up. The other key is your body. You have to take control of your medications to make sure they're in the right balance for you."

"But *when* will I feel better?" he pressed.

"You will feel better," I said, "as your mind and body get healthier. You will recover, but you will have to learn not to depend so much on others. You will have to get better by yourself, for yourself, on your own."

Today, Cojo is doing well with his second transplanted kidney. Sandra is doing well with Ernesto's kidney. And I am doing well with Gregg's kidney. We all survived.

Many Americans who suffer from organ failure do not survive. Recall that the number who die while waiting for a transplant is about 6,500 per year, or 18 people each day. These are people whose lives could have been saved. But despite all the battles between the Free Market Camp and the Human Rights Camp, all the literature on the ethical and religious and social problems—all those nasty collisions between economics, politics, and law—America's organ transplant policy remains fatally flawed. It is time for meaningful change.

PART THREE

THE SEARCH
FOR SOLUTIONS

CHAPTER ELEVEN

THE BAND-AID APPROACH

Remember the "kidney swap" performed by Dr. Zaki Shapira in Tel Aviv? The one where a Jewish man from Jerusalem suffered from kidney failure but couldn't use his wife's kidney because she was not a match, and an Arab woman from a village near Haifa suffering from kidney damage couldn't use her husband's kidney because he was not a match? Dr. Shapira figured out that the Jewish woman was a good match for the Arab woman and the Arab guy was a good match for the Jewish guy. The two transplants were performed in tandem at the same hospital, and Dr. Shapira was lauded for it in the Arab press. In the context of his shady exploits in the organ markets, however, these early kidney swaps suffered from guilt by association.

If the infamous organ outlaw was doing it, it couldn't be good. Could it?

Well, it's happened here in America! The National Organ Transplant Act (NOTA) was amended in December 2007 to allow the friends and families of patients in need of organ transplants to bring together the families and friends of other patients on the waiting list to save lives through organ swaps. It is called human organ paired donation.[1]

The story of this new law—the Charlie W. Norwood Living Organ Donation Act—demonstrates two things: Where there is a political will, there is a way, and modest efforts to expand the availability of organs are not enough. The story likely begins in places like Israel, where people like Zaki Shapira started performing the swaps, usually simultaneously in the same hospital.

Then, in 2004, the *New York Times* reported a privately arranged kidney swap in America that followed the pattern.[2] Enter Charlie Norwood, the Republican congressman from Georgia.[3] A dentist and Vietnam vet, he was a staunch conservative when it came to immigration control, and he opposed renewal of the Voting Rights Act because, he said, it discriminated against southern states for wrongs remedied long ago. But Norwood was liberal when it came to things like patients' rights. Maybe that's because he suffered from idiopathic pulmonary fibrosis and had a lung transplant in 2004. Less than 2 years after that, after having a cancerous tumor removed from his lung, he started chemotherapy for liver cancer; the cancers were thought to have been caused by the immunosuppressant drugs he had to take after his lung transplant.

Norwood introduced legislation to amend NOTA to allow organ swaps in early 2007. He died shortly thereafter. His bill was passed unanimously by the Senate and overwhelmingly by the House, and it was signed by President George W. Bush in late December.[4] Along the way, it was renamed for its sponsor. The statute makes it clear that NOTA's prohibition against the buying and selling of transplant organs "does not apply with respect to human organ paired donation."

Then the statute defines "human organ paired donation" as the donation and receipt of human organs under these circumstances:[5]

(A) An individual (referred to in this paragraph as the "first donor") desires to make a living donation of a human organ specifically to a particular patient (referred to in this paragraph as the "first patient"), but such donor is biologically incompatible as a donor for such patient.

(B) A second individual (referred to in this paragraph as the "second donor") desires to make a living donation of a human organ specifically to a second particular patient (referred to in this paragraph as the "second patient"), but such donor is biologically incompatible as a donor for such patient.

(C) Subject to subparagraph (D), the first donor is biologically compatible as a donor of a human organ for the second patient, and the second donor is biologically compatible as a donor of a human organ for the first patient.

(D) If there is any additional donor-patient pair as described in subparagraph (A) or (B), each donor in the group of donor-patient pairs is biologically compatible as a donor of a human organ for a patient in such group.

(E) All donors and patients in the group of donor-patient pairs (whether 2 pairs or more than 2 pairs) enter into a single agreement to donate and receive such human organs, respectively, according to such biological compatibility in the group.

(F) Other than as described in subparagraph (E), no valuable consideration is knowingly acquired, received, or otherwise transferred with respect to the human organs referred to in such subparagraph.

Carl Levin, the Democrat from Michigan who sponsored the bill in the Senate, explained it this way:[6]

> Our legislation . . . will save lives by increasing the number of kidneys available for transplantation. . . . It addresses [a] relatively new procedure, which is supported by numerous medical organizations, including the United Network for Organ Sharing, the American Society of Transplant

Surgeons, the American Society of Transplantation, the National Kidney Foundation and the American Society of Pediatric Nephrology. Paired organ donation, which did not exist when [NOTA] was enacted more than two decades ago, will make it possible for thousands of people who wish to donate a kidney to a spouse, family member or friend, but find that they are medically incompatible, to still become living kidney donors.

The legislation is necessary because [NOTA], which contains a prohibition intended by Congress to preclude purchasing organs, is unintentionally impeding the facilitation of matching incompatible pairs. Our legislation would simply add kidney paired donation to the list of other living-related donation exemptions that Congress originally placed in NOTA. It removes an unintended impediment to kidney paired donations by clarifying ambiguous language in Section 301 of [NOTA]. That section has been interpreted by a number of Transplant Centers to prohibit such donations. . . .

Congress surely never intended that the living donation arrangements that permit kidney paired donation be impeded by NOTA. Our bill simply makes that clear. Some transplant professionals involved in these and other innovative living kidney donation arrangements have proceeded in the reasonable belief that these arrangements do not violate Section 301 of NOTA, but they contend that they are doing so under a cloud.

And exactly what is the nature of the cloud that had to be removed?

It's the fact that NOTA prohibits the payment of "valuable consideration" for a transplant organ, and "valuable consideration" is not limited, according to universal legal interpretation, to the exchange of money. Under basic contract law, a promise for a promise will do. Thus, organ swaps by definition involve valuable consideration: The first patient only gets an organ because the second patient gets one. One is the condition to the other. The new law removes this cloud by exempting swaps from the definition. Curiously, subparagraphs D and E seem to go further in allowing types of swaps that involve more than the original four-person configuration. For example, does the new legislation authorize organizations like LifeSharers,[7] which promotes a member-based version of the concept? Those who join LifeSharers agree to donate their organs to other members. Should a member need an organ, like nonmembers, he or she begins the process by getting on the United Network for Organ Sharing (UNOS) waiting list. If, however, a LifeSharers member dies with organs eligible for transplantation, the LifeSharers member highest on the waiting list is supposed to get access to those organs before any nonmembers. UNOS has not challenged the group, though its ethics committee originally "declined to offer support."[8]

Other issues that are not addressed by the new law will have to be resolved as people push the limits of the process. The statute does not, for example, require that paired donations occur simultaneously, let alone in the same hospital. What if the first transplant goes forward but the second is stalled because the second donor changes his or her mind? Would an American court actually force a person to go under the knife in order to enforce the bargain? These questions are hardly fanciful given the language of the law. But more importantly, how significant an impact has the new law had? The waiting lists are longer than ever. So far, the impact of the new amendment has been minimal.

And that's typical of federal initiatives when it comes to organ transplant reform. On April 5, 2004, President Bush signed the Organ Donation and Recovery Improvement Act, which authorized a paltry amount, only $25 million over 5 years, for grants designed to stimulate organ availability—mostly through donor awareness programs—as well as more limited grants for reimbursement of the subsistence and travel expenses incurred by live organ donors.[9] Four years later, the funding for this exceedingly modest program still had not been appropriated![10]

Meanwhile, in July 2004, UNOS issued two new policies: "Organ Procurement, Distribution and Allocation" and "Allocation of Deceased Kidneys."[11] They were long and technical. The new rules on kidney allocation expanded the criteria governing donors based on cause of death, history of hypertension, and creatinine levels. The formulas were absolutely mind-boggling. A system based on "time of waiting points," antigen mismatch, panel reactive antibody levels, and medical urgency was detailed.

Then, in November 2004, UNOS issued a press release opposing solicitation for organs when no personal bond existed between the patient and the donor or his family.[12] "'Organ donation is a gift, not a transaction,'" said UNOS president Robert Metzger, MD. "'[W]e strongly oppose public or private appeals that effectively put the needs of one candidate above all others and pose concerns of fairness.' . . . [T]he OPTN system is designed to allocate organs equitably according to the greatest need and/or benefit of all candidates."

UNOS continues to revise its policies concerning organ allocation. Throughout 2007 it issued a virtual tsunami of proposals and guidelines designed to improve the existing system.[13] Special attention was paid to standards governing live organ donations and the securing of proper consent from live donors. The walls of the transplant maze grew thicker and the path seemed more treacherous than ever.

Finally, late in 2007, UNOS dropped a bombshell. It floated the idea of moving away from a system based on the time a patient spends waiting on the list to a system based on which patients can best use the organs that are available. UNOS argued that the new system would make more efficient use of organs by lessening the chance of rejection. It acknowledged, however, that the new system would also disadvantage those who had waited longest on the lists, mostly older patients. The proposal prompted a lively debate on Minnesota Public Radio.[14]

What is important is this: The UNOS proposals address the subject of organ allocation within the existing statutory framework: how to best use the organs that are available rather than how to increase the pool of donors. Increasing the pool of donors has largely been left to the states and, for the most part, their efforts have been modest—providing small tax and insurance incentives, funding donor awareness programs, and making access to donor registration forms easier.

The Charlie W. Norwood Living Organ Donation Act proves this point. It is modest in its impact at best. It is designed to make more transplants available without truly increasing the pool of already-willing donors. In other words, it seeks to improve the efficiency of organ allocation. It does not seek to effect deep reform.

We have to look elsewhere to find innovation.

Brad is the youngest of my three sons. He is handsome like Gregg and Brent, a smart kid who recently graduated from Yeshiva University's Benjamin N. Cardozo School of Law in New York and now works in Washington, DC. Because he is the youngest, Brad claims Cindy and I were always more lenient with him.

Brad first learned of my kidney problems after my physical early in the summer of 2003. I sat my entire family down in the breakfast room of our home in Denver and told them what the doctors were saying. The idea of a transplant at the time was very abstract. It was only a distant possibility.

After a trip through Europe with his cousin that summer, Brad returned home to find me considerably slowed down. In August, he went with me and my entourage to Johns Hopkins to hear our fears confirmed. Later that same month, Brad, Brent, Gregg, and I traveled to Las Vegas for the bachelor party for Norm Brownstein's son.

I was staying with my friends at the Mirage and the younger guys were staying with their friends at the Hard Rock. I called my sons and asked them to come over to the Mirage to talk. On a steaming summer day in the desert, we sat in the air-conditioned living room of my suite overlooking the Strip. Waves of heat shimmered outside.

I started talking to my three sons: "I've lived a good life, but how much longer I'll have to live it—"

They immediately interrupted me. Brad recalls that it was like I was speaking my last words to them. It really hit home. It was like a farewell.

"No," insisted all three sons, "you'll be fine. You have plenty more years."

"Don't say that," I said. "We don't know if it's true."

Everyone fell silent. A few more sentences were exchanged, but mostly it was quiet—and gloomy. This meeting, he says, put it all in perspective. He went back to college in the fall and prepared to graduate in the spring. He was slated to move to Washington to take an internship with Senate Minority Leader Tom Daschle before moving to New York to start law school.

Everything was laid out for him. Everything but his father.

"It was late September, maybe early October," Brad recalls, "when I contacted Tara Morgan, my dad's transplant caseworker at the University of Colorado. I told her I would be willing to donate my kidney to my dad. After that, I had my blood taken and I answered some questions. But it never went any further than that. I never got a call back to take the tests to the next step."

Brad wondered why until he learned Cindy had called Tara and told her to take him off the possible donor list. He was angry and disappointed when he learned of her intervention—"He's not old enough," Cindy had insisted—but he understood. Brad says, "Tara knew what my mom was going through and she didn't want to make matters any worse. The fact that my mother was in denial doesn't mean she wasn't active or involved."

What kept Brad off the list was Cindy's effective veto power. He encountered a form of the "family veto." This is a practical term of art used throughout the transplant community. It is not, however, a legal term. Brad's encounter occurred in connection with a possible live organ donation. More often, the family veto is used to keep a deceased donor's organs from being taken, even if he or she has registered as an organ donor and made his or her wish to donate clear.

Despite recent efforts to negate the family veto through revisions to the Uniform Anatomical Gift Act (UAGA), most doctors agree that it remains a problem that limits the use of available organs. I do not believe that it should be allowed to frustrate the wishes of a competent adult who has expressed his or her wishes in an organ donor registry, living will, driver's license form, or other legally cognizable way. Yet fear of liability, respect for family wishes, and continued lack of specificity in the UAGA prevent health care professionals from doing all they can to harvest all the available organs.

The original UAGA was drafted in 1968 by the National Conference of Commissioners on Uniform State Laws. In 1987, it was amended to provide that an "anatomical gift that is not revoked by the donor before death is irrevocable and does not require the consent or concurrence of any person after the donor's death."[15] The amendment was meant to make clear that "consent of next of kin after death is not required." The amendment failed in its intent for a number of reasons.

First, the UAGA had to be adopted by each state individually. Colorado did not, for example, adopt the new language until 1998.[16] Second, the language of the amendment merely authorized the harvesting of organs without family consent. It did not require that health care professionals carry out the donor's intent, nor did it forbid consultation with the family. Third, not every state adopted the language of the amendment as written. Maine, for example, passed a statute in 2003 that provided simple procedures whereby the "next of kin to a person who has expressed intent to donate that person's own body organs or tissue after death may override the intention of the donor."[17]

Then there were the lawsuits. In December 2004, the *Portland Press Herald and Maine Sunday Telegram* reported on several lawsuits filed in Maine, Massachusetts, Virginia, and Missouri alleging the wrongful taking of organs.[18] Suits like these, and others that have been filed more recently, have deterred health care professionals from doing everything possible to carry out the clear wishes of deceased donors.

Plainly, the 1987 amendments to the UAGA did not, in practice, go far enough in negating the family veto. The National Kidney Foundation has estimated that up to one-third of the kidneys that could have been harvested from deceased donors who had indicated their desire to donate were not used to avoid violating the families' wishes.

So in 2006 and 2007, a whole new Revised UAGA was presented

to the states.[19] Like the earlier versions, it must be adopted by each state individually. And it continues to prohibit the buying and selling of organs: "A person that for valuable consideration, knowingly purchases or sells a part for transplantation or therapy if removal of a part from an individual is intended to occur after the individual's death commits a [felony]."

Included are detailed provisions designed to make the donation process clearer and more efficient at the operational level. And one more stab is taken at negating the family veto: "[I]n the absence of an express, contrary indication by the donor, a person other than the donor is barred from making, amending, or revoking an anatomical gift of a donor's body or part if the donor made an anatomical gift of the donor's body or part" in accordance with the statute.[20]

What could possibly be clearer than that?

Anecdotally, according to Dr. Kam, despite the clear intent and language of the new statute, doctors still ask the family for permission to harvest a loved one's organs. They usually refrain from taking the deceased's organs if the family strongly objects. What this shows is simple, and it is the same lesson my son Brad learned: At difficult emotional times, the wishes of the family will often override, however informally but effectively, the wishes of the donor and the dictates of the law.

To correct this situation we must address the dynamics of the family. At the most basic level, we need to learn to talk about these life-and-death decisions. So many of the difficulties I faced during my transplant adventure stemmed from Cindy's and others' unwillingness to talk openly about my dilemmas. Denial ran rampant. The solution seemed so simple and so obvious: Talk about it! But so few people wanted to.

How many people make their wishes about their willingness to donate their organs clearly known? This is not something people talk about unless it's in the context of a big news story like the Terri Schiavo case.[21] Think how much time, effort, money, emotional turmoil, media coverage, and political posturing could have been saved if only Terri Schiavo had simply made her wishes clearly known? Her husband and friends all agreed that she had said she would not want to live in a vegetative state. Yet her mother, father, and siblings insisted that she would want to fight for every breath of life, however artificially induced. Whose position would rule the day?

Would it not have been so much better if Terri Schiavo had talked explicitly about her wishes—and put them in writing: What sorts of extraordinary medical efforts would she want to keep her alive? When should attempts be made to resuscitate her if she expired? Did she wish to donate her organs? All of them, or just some of them?

Adults are responsible for making their wishes known. And adults should take the next step: Sign the necessary documents. If people really want to make their wishes known and avoid arguments at delicate times, then they must put them in writing. It's best if they execute both testamentary wills and living wills. Even if they do not, they should register as organ donors. Sign their driver's license organ donor forms. Do whatever it takes under their states' laws to make their wishes clear and legally enforceable.

If you walk into the emergency room in many hospitals today, you are handed a 12-page document called "Five Wishes." It asks: Who do you want to make health care decisions for you when you can't make them for yourself? What kinds of medical treatments do or don't you want? How comfortable do you wish to be made? How do you want people to treat you? What do you want your loved ones to know?

The Five Wishes is a voluntary project created by a nonprofit entity called Aging with Dignity.[22] Hospitals are not required to participate. The "Five Wishes" document addresses most of the questions raised by the Schiavo case and more. It provides for execution with the formalities required to be legally enforceable in most states. But it barely addresses organ donation. Amid the details in the 12 pages, only two short sentences address that subject. On page 5, you are given the choice of authorizing your "health care agent" to "donate useable organs or tissues of mine as allowed by law." And on page 9, the form asks "for any other wishes. For example, you may want to donate any or all parts of your body when you die."

In other words, while trying to tackle the really big taboos—those tough decisions many face at the end of life—"Five Wishes" leaves out any practically usable detail on donating your organs. The solution is simple: Add a "Sixth Wish" to address clearly and legally what your wishes are with respect to organ and tissue donation. Only then should the document be called complete.

Simply put, we just don't talk about it enough or sign enough documents to make our wishes clear. Even when we do, as a practical matter, doctors still most often seek consent from the family before harvesting organs from a loved one. Why? The reasons are partly medical. It's because, as Dr. Chan once explained to me, most of today's forms that address organ donation presume you're already dead or at least brain-dead. Optimal use of your organs, however, often requires that basic tests be run before death or brain death. Whether they are legally required to or not, doctors typically respect the wishes of the family as long as you are alive. Therefore, your desire to donate could be frustrated by medical decisions—like a spouse withholding consent for those pretransplant tests—made while you are still technically living.

The Revised UAGA still does not go far enough in negating family vetoes. Even to the extent that it succeeds, it simply makes available organs that the donors were already willing to give. In this way, it is much like the recent amendments to NOTA that authorize kidney swaps: Both statutes increase the number of transplants by making better use of already available organs rather than by significantly expanding the donor pool.

Legislation that does try to increase the number of willing donors has, however, been introduced in many states. These proposals come in many sizes and flavors. They start with this reality: Supply does not meet demand under any of the current approaches. And the gap is getting wider. Not enough people who are willing to donate organs leave wills or living wills to declare their gifts. Not enough people check the little boxes on their driver's license forms to consent to donating their organs upon death. Not enough families donate the organs of their deceased loved ones. And not enough doctors ask families to donate the organs of their loved ones.

Ironically, observes one writer, advances in medicine have contributed to America's organ shortage.[23] Great strides in the practice of organ transplantation have resulted in its widespread use. The advent of "life-maintenance equipment such as respirators, ventilators, and dialysis machines" has increased the number of people who survive serious illnesses and need organ transplants. The development of powerful immunosuppressant drugs has helped control rejection of transplantable organs. Advances like these have made transplants routine, inhibited only by the lack of organs.

Modest proposals to increase the pool of donors work within the present system. In 1994, Pennsylvania created an Organ Donation Awareness Trust Fund.[24] Under the plan, the state department of health receives the funds when Pennsylvanians choose to contribute $1 upon renewing their driver's licenses, registering their vehicles, or filing their state income tax returns. Up to 10 percent of the funds may be used each year for the reasonable medical expenses of donors, "paid to the funeral home or hospital, but not to the donor's family or estate." The statute allows payments of up to $3,000 per family, but the committee that administers the plan has, so far, set the payment levels much lower.

Yet even this modest plan received a mixed response.[25] The past president of the Transplant Recipients International Organization called the plan "very dangerous," and Francis Delmonico, MD, director of the kidney transplant program at Massachusetts General Hospital, declared that "society is not prepared to allow for your body to be bought and sold." Representatives from the federal government warned that the Pennsylvania plan would require "close scrutiny to determine if it violates the 1984 transplantation law."

Despite these warnings, many other states have tried to stimulate organ donation. A majority have expanded their laws concerning medical leaves to accommodate and encourage transplants. In Michigan, legislation has been introduced that would give living donors, in the year of their donation, a credit of up to $10,000 against their income for tax purposes.[26] Similar tax credit legislation has been proposed at the federal level.

What all of these proposals have in common is this: They are only modest responses to major problems. They tinker with the system without deeply reforming it. They may well cause marginal increases in the donor pool, but they do not pack enough punch to really reduce the waiting lists.

What more can be done? Two suggestions are offered in the next chapter. First, however, let us consider two proposals that likely cannot be adopted in America today. No, not the harvesting of organs from executed prisoners, like they used to do in China. While some have proposed that solution in our country, no one takes them seriously.[27] What we need to address are proposals for the replacement of our "opt-in" system with an "opt-out" or presumed consent system and the adoption of free markets in organs in America. Legislation that was introduced in Delaware in January 2008 to adopt an "opt-out" system in that state is already making waves in the transplant community.[28]

In 1986, the Florida Supreme Court upheld an early presumed consent statute that allowed the removal of corneas even against the wishes of the deceased's family.[29] The United States Supreme Court has declined to review limited laws similar to these.[30] But in January 2008, legislation to adopt an opt-out system in Delaware was introduced by state representative Pete Schwartzkopf, who donated a kidney to a friend in 2006.[31]

"It's going to change the way we do organ donation in our state," he said.

Forget the abuses of opt-out systems in Third World countries like Brazil, where local corruption can be blamed. The inspiration for the bill that would make Delaware the first state to apply presumed consent to vital organs, rather than only to tissues like corneas, came to Schwartzkopf from Europe. Austria, Spain, Portugal, Italy, Belgium, Bulgaria, France, Luxembourg, Norway, Finland, Sweden, Switzerland, Latvia, the Czech Republic, the Slovak Republic, Hungary, Slovenia, Poland, Greece, and Singapore all have some form of opt-out or presumed consent system.

In January 2008, British prime minister Gordon Brown called for his country's adoption of a presumed consent system.[32] The British press responded with enthusiastic support. Commentators from the *Observer* announced a "revolution in the way organs are donated for transplant."

Why wouldn't an opt-out or presumed consent system work here in America? Well, it turns out that the system does not really help that much. European countries still suffer from dramatic shortages of organs.

According to a 2005 study by Kieran Healy from the University of Arizona, "Countries with presumed consent laws are found to have higher procurement rates, but the effect is relatively weak. Evidence from two presumed-consent counties where procurement rates have grown rapidly (Spain and Italy) suggests that the legal regime is a marker for other organizational practices rather than a causal mechanism in itself. More broadly, donor procurement takes place within societies that have institutionalized different relationships between the individual, the market, and the state. . . . [L]iberal regimes always have informed consent rules."[33] Huh?

What this means is that presumed consent in itself doesn't boost procurement rates that much. Most estimate that it's by less than 15 to 20 percent. And in Spain and Italy, where procurement rates are notably higher, other factors influence donation as much as if not more than the legality of the opt-out system. These additional factors include more public education about donation and transplantation, appeals to ethics and charity, vigorous encouragement of donation by the Catholic Church, clinical practices that enhance the harvesting of organs, and the social welfare environment. A June 2007 analysis of presumed consent legislation across Europe found that "a wealthy, dominantly Catholic presumed consent country with greater civil liberties is more likely to have higher cadaveric donation rates [but] a larger potential pool of organs is more effective to combat organ shortage in wealthy informed consent countries."[34]

Here in the United States, our doctors have a hard enough time disregarding the family veto. Imagine if they had to enforce an opt-out system. Our basic ideas, both constitutional and political, about self-autonomy and the integrity of the body stand as a roadblock to a universal presumed consent system in the United States.

Is this roadblock insurmountable?

For the near future, the answer is probably yes. The "professional consensus," according to the Prefatory Note to the Revised UAGA, "appears to be not to replace the present opt-in principle at this time." If the medical establishment is not behind a move to presumed consent in America, it is hard to see how such an important change could be made. So much of our legal and medical system is based on that common law concept of "informed consent," and nothing flies in the face of informed consent more than presumed consent. You can't really have both.

Indiana law professor David Orentlicher, MD, in a forthcoming *Rutgers Law Review* article, "Presumed Consent to Organ Donation: Its Rise and Fall in the United States," explains why the movement fizzled.[35] There were several reasons: Because "it could not overcome the major reason why people do not become organ donors after death—the refusal of family members to give consent to donation. To the extent that presumed consent allowed family members to overcome the presumption and withhold consent, it did not address the reasons why family members say no. [And to] the extent that professionals tried to preserve the presumption by bypassing families, they validated fears that doctors will be too quick to take organs from dead persons who would not have wanted their organs removed. . . . [O]ther proposed reforms will be needed to address the shortage of organs for transplantation."

And that's without talking about the actual mechanics of the opt-out system. Most people in the United States do not get that far. It is one thing to encourage donation. It is another thing to force it.

Those Supreme Court cases that enshrine the rights of privacy and self-autonomy, protecting the personal nature of decisions about the most intimate bodily matters, would most likely invalidate all but the most narrowly tailored presumed consent laws applying to organs. At the very least, the ability to opt out would have to be made easily and lavishly available.

On balance, it appears that widespread adoption of presumed

consent laws in America is not likely. These laws do not dramatically increase organ donation rates unless they are strictly enforced and accompanied by additional procurement efforts, they violate long-standing traditions grounded in the idea of informed consent, and they might well violate the constitutional right of privacy. While Delaware's pending law might trigger a revolution, it's unlikely that America will opt in to opt out in the near future. Its benefits simply are not significant enough to make it a compelling alternative.

Like kidney swaps and the Revised UAGA, it is just another Band-Aid.

I celebrated the 1st anniversary of my transplant in Prague. Cindy and I were traveling with two other couples from Denver. We had just visited Warsaw, and Vienna was next on our itinerary. I was feeling contemplative, thinking about really big issues—issues of life and death—evoked by our tour of the Warsaw Ghetto. From there, millions of Polish Jews were shipped to Auschwitz and other Nazi extermination camps.

Before World War II, one in every three Poles was Jewish. Three million in a country of 9 million. Today, there are 3,000 Jews in Poland. Dealing with all that conflict—the sheer magnitude of it—was occupying my thoughts during that part of the trip. Also, Warsaw was where Jews had mounted a massive though unsuccessful revolt against the Nazis. So I was also thinking about bravery and the Masada complex, which holds that fighting to the end is preferable to surrender. I remembered how Jewish rebels held out against Roman legions at Masada during ancient times. And how, eventually, they all committed suicide rather than being taken alive. Well, the uprising in the Warsaw Ghetto was a lot like that.

And all that death makes you appreciate life. When we went to the train tracks where the Nazis herded the Jews—and gypsies and gays—onto cars destined to take them to their deaths, Cindy's face turned ashen. She said she would have killed herself before she ever would have gotten on the train. I was feeling feisty and strong by then. I boasted, "I wouldn't have let you. I would have protected you. And I would have led the revolt!"

Then I found myself in Prague, on the anniversary of my transplant, shopping for Bohemian crystal on the second floor of Moser Glass, thinking again about life and death. But not, ironically, about the day of my surgery. In fact, I did not think about that until much later that night. By then the Old Town Square was packed. A hundred thousand people had come to listen to rock bands and watch the Czech hockey team play for the World Cup on giant video screens.

We strolled from the Four Seasons, only a couple of blocks from all that noise, across the Charles Bridge. Street artists and musicians plied their wares every few steps, and tourists weaved their way through the throngs. The giant Castle of Prague loomed black and crenellated and scary over us. We ate dinner at a place called Kampa Park, nestled on the bank of the Vltava River, at the base of the bridge.

Finally I put it all together, that fierce attachment to life evoked by our visit to the Warsaw Ghetto, amplified by the 1st anniversary of my surgery. I offered a champagne toast to the occasion. It was the first drink of alcohol I had taken in more than a year.

After visiting Prague we went to Vienna. Our guide in Prague put us in touch with a government official in Vienna who was Jewish and willing to talk about Jewish life in Austria. We bought him lunch at an Italian restaurant. He was in his fifties and had lived in Vienna most of his life. He told us there were 200,000 Jews in Austria before World War II, and now there are only 3,000.

Were all the others killed in the war? No, explained our lunch guest, many converted to Christianity and survived. Austrian Jews, he said, were never like those who shut themselves into ghettos. They were secular people outside their private lives. They maintained their Jewish identities in little "study rooms" while they assimilated.

And so I pondered not only death, but the death of my people, the Jewish people: the disappearing Jew.

It was nothing new. After the Spanish Expulsion in 1492, many Jews converted to Christianity rather than leave their homes. Many of these so-called conversos continued to practice their Jewish religion secretly and became known as crypto-Jews or Marranos— "pigs" in Spanish. They were targets in the Spanish Inquisition, for the Catholic Church did not have authority over Jews who simply overstayed their welcome in Spain. That was purely a civil matter. But apostasy was a matter for the priests.

So the idea of converting to stay alive during the war was familiar to the Jews. Our guide in Vienna was a blonde, blue-eyed woman. She told us that when her father died at the age of 90, her aunt—his sister—told her, for the first time, that their family had Jewish blood. Today, there are only 13 million Jews left in the world. There are hundreds of millions—billions, even—of members of the other major religions: Islam, Christianity, Hindu, and Buddhism. But only 13 million Jews, half of whom live in a country less than 60 years old and in a constant state of conflict.

I said to myself, after listening to our guest and our guide, *Boy, the things people will do to stay alive.* And of course that included the things I had done—the kidney I had taken from my own son—to stay alive myself. The transplant experience, for me, had finally brought together the material and the spiritual worlds. I saw that life occurs whenever they come together. And death occurs when they separate.

I remember thinking, there in Vienna, about a speech given by Pope John Paul II in 1993, when he came to Denver to celebrate World Youth Day.[36] He had chosen Denver as the place to deliver his message to a global audience of young people, says one writer, "precisely because of Denver's secularity, its self-conscious modernity, and its sense of living on the cutting edge of the high tech future."

It was August 12 and very hot and dry when two Boeing 747s touched down at Stapleton International Airport. The first was *Air Force One*. I greeted Bill Clinton when he got off the plane, and later that night we hosted a fund-raiser for Colorado governor Roy Romer in that big United Airlines hangar they had at the old airport. When I introduced President Clinton to the crowd, I joked, "A year before last November's election, if you had told me that we would be electing a Democrat from Arkansas as our new president, I'd have said, 'Sure, and the pope will be coming to Denver.' Well, we did elect a Democrat from Arkansas, and today, the pope has come to Denver!"

The second Boeing 747 that touched down at Stapleton that Thursday afternoon was an Alitalia with Vatican markings. We watched as the pope came down the ramp in his Pope-mobile. Already you could tell he was getting old, and his Parkinson's disease was showing. He looked frail. But he had such an incredible presence. And Denver went completely wild. Vendors sold Pope-on-a-Rope on the Sixteenth Street Mall. That's right: soap on a rope in the shape of the pope! Renters paid incredible premiums for housing near the pontiff's appearances. He packed 90,000 into Mile High Stadium. More than 200,000 young people from all over the world came to Denver to hear him speak.

A quarter of a million toting sleeping bags, water bottles, and backpacks hiked the 15 miles from downtown to Cherry Creek State Park on Saturday. That night, the pope gave a speech to them. His words evoked many of the themes I have encountered on my transplant journey. He said to the youth, "In the modern metropolis . . . , life is often treated as just one more commodity to be organized, commercialized and manipulated according to convenience . . . The drama of the moral crisis of modernity was that so many people refused to recognize the threat posed to life by reducing it to a commodity."

I guess that says it all: That's the reason it is so unlikely that free markets in human transplant organs will be allowed in America in the near future. We simply are not ready to take that step, no matter how alluring the logic and economics appear to be.

Assume, for the moment, that the economists and the bloggers are right. Many of the problems with organ markets in Third World countries would not arise here in America. Those problems that do arise could be handled with mild regulation. The risk of complications or death for live organ donors in America is less than 0.1 percent. And legally, shouldn't we be able to do what we want, within reason, with our own bodies, according to the right to privacy and all that?

There it is again, the link between economics and law. We might as well add politics, because in this case the three of them conspire to doom organ markets in America in the near future. Start with the simple reality that every Western democratic country prohibits the buying and selling of organs. The list of opponents is growing as nations like China and India at least formally adopt bans on the illicit trade. We are not likely to join Iran as the second country in the world to adopt a market system. And, even then, the Iranian system is not a truly free market, but rather a very heavily regulated market.

America would adopt an opt-out presumed consent system, with all of its flaws and limitations, before it would adopt free markets in organs. The relationship between such markets and the internal political processes in emerging nations was the key to their original growth abroad. When Dr. Nancy Scheper-Hughes conducted her initial research in Brazil and Argentina, she found in these Latin American countries that "the organ stealing rumors surfaced during or soon after the democratization process was initiated and in the wake of human rights reports."[37] Again we see the strong connection between commerce in organs and the forces of globalization, democratization, and the rule of law.

Dr. Scheper-Hughes also said, "Under apartheid and under South Africa's new, democratic, and neo-liberal context, organ transplant practices reveal the marked social and economic cleavages that separate donors and recipients into two opposed and antagonistic populations."[38] She summarized the South African case this way: "As organ transplantation moves into the private sector, commercialism has taken hold. In the absence of a national policy regulating transplant surgery and no regional, let alone national, official waiting lists, the distribution of transplantable organs is informal and subject to corruption."[39]

Let's just face it. These conditions do not exist in America. We are unlikely to emulate the primitive systems of emerging countries. No, in the United States, the free markets in organs would be more sophisticated. Fifteen years ago, Gloria Banks described the major types of proposed regulated systems for the transplant industry: the living provider organ market, the posthumous organ market, and the combined altruistic/commercial organ market.[40]

Banks concluded, "In light of the ethical and legal issues raised thus far, a combined altruistic/posthumous commercial organ market provides the most viable solution to the ongoing shortage of human organs for transplant purposes. The other systems require more extensive ethical and legal safeguards to protect vulnerable citizens and are unlikely to overcome the major arguments raised against the commercialization of human organs."

To regulate these markets, Banks set out safeguards:[41]

(1) "noncompulsory participation" in order to satisfy the informed consent doctrine

(2) "preservation of the states' interest in protecting human life" in cases of incompetence

(3) "retirement of social worth valuations" to avoid the worst abuses associated with organ markets, namely "society's attempt to make human life valuations based on an individual's perceived social worth"

(4) "retention of a nonprofit-making and noncompetitive market system" so not all eggs are placed in the commercialization basket

Shaun Pattinson of the Sheffield Institute of Biotechnological Law and Ethics in England similarly argues for "regulated commercial dealings in organs from live organ providers."[42] He says that many "regulatory safeguards are capable of applying to living organ providers, including the imposition of compulsory waiting periods between agreeing to sell and organ removal, a minimum age of the seller, a minimum price mechanism, preoperative assessment panels (including, say, physicians and social workers), the imposition of mandatory financial disclosure and counseling requirements, restrictions on those able to buy organs, the separation of buying and allocation bodies, and the restriction of the commercial market to particular jurisdictions."

The list of limitations and regulations for the proposed organ markets grows. The maze becomes impenetrable. None of the Band-Aid solutions solves the problem. Could we as a people accept the moral and ethical consequences of adopting truly free markets in organs? Some argue that the ethics involved are different than those in other situations where bodies have been commodified. Pointing to the involuntary nature of slavery, they distinguish the precedents that give our hearts pause.

But I do not buy it. It won't happen in America in the near future. So if free markets are too extreme and presumed consent is insufficiently effective, what can we really do?

CHAPTER TWELVE

THE REALITIES OF REFORM

I celebrated the 1-year anniversary of my transplant in Prague, thinking about life and death. Ernesto Delaroca spent the day in Denver, working as usual. He didn't recall the day was special until he was reminded. He didn't think about life and death. But that night he feasted, as well. He and his family had spent the prior weekend camping and fishing in western Nebraska, and Ernesto had caught a big white bass.

On May 11, 2005, Ernesto's wife, Gicela, served homemade tortillas and fish stew made with that white bass. Ernesto may have been born a peasant, but that night he ate like a king. He looked across the table and smiled at Sandra, healthy again, thank God.

She'd been only 18 when she had first heard him tell how the right-wing death squad had burst into their home and dragged their parents into the night. Now, she'd had 4 years to think about it—with kidney failure and a transplant in between.

Sandra knew that if she were still living in Guatemala—well, she knew she would not still be living in Guatemala. Having survived her family's political tragedy in 1984, she most certainly would have died from her medical condition. The public health system in Guatemala was primitive at best, especially in rural places. Sandra could neither have afforded nor obtained a kidney transplant in her native land. But here in the United States, she had received the medical services—courtesy of its limited public insurance programs—that allowed her to take Ernesto's kidney.

Like me, she was a recipient. A lot of the flowers she saw when she woke up at University Hospital had come from my room down the hall. Her brother, Ernesto, and my son Gregg became heroes. I took home awards. What became of Sandra?

She was still living with Ernesto and his family in a small, blond brick house in Lakewood, a downscale suburb west of Denver. It wasn't the same house where Ernesto had first told the tale of his parents' disappearance. That house had been a rental. This one had been purchased by the Delarocas with hard work and hard-earned American dollars.

It was much more to them than bricks. To them, it was the American dream come true. On the porch, a series of seats covered in blankets faced West Colorado Drive. In the tiny garden between the front porch and the close-cropped yard, flowers bloomed. An older Chevy pickup was parked at the curb. It was black and rusted and had a snowplow affixed to the front. In the open-sided carport, a newer purple Toyota pickup—Ernesto's pickup—sat next to Gali's pink scooter with its little pink basket. It was a setting many Americans would have viewed as lower class or lower middle class at best.

To Sandra, it was paradise. A year after receiving Ernesto's kidney she was still shy, but had grown quick to laugh. Her mood was cheerful. Her English was still limited and her Spanish came in rapid-fire bursts, punctuated with the giggles of a girl. She had blonde streaks in her dark hair and liked to listen to music, especially hip-hop and rock, especially the group Gasoline.

In other words, a year after receiving Ernesto's kidney, Sandra was feeling great. She was working at Wendy's 40 hours a week and liked her job. She did not have a boyfriend—giggle, giggle—but dreamed about having a family of her own someday. She'd gone from taking 14 different prescription drugs each day to 5. The drugs still affected her activity level—they made her sleepy and unable to drive—so she looked forward to taking less. After dinner that night, she sat on the couch and twirled the remote to the big-screen TV that dominated the living room.

Sandra and I have never met, not before our surgeries or since. She has never met Jim Sullivan, Ernesto's former employer, though she has met his brother Pat, who speaks fluent Spanish, and Jim's wife, Lynne, who had taken a lot of my flowers down the hall to her room. Thinking back, 1 year after the surgery, Sandra realized she had never even asked where all those flowers had come from. She did know she had been able to leave the hospital before the "important man" down the hall.

Today, when asked if she would ever like to go back to Guatemala, Sandra shakes her head emphatically and says, "No." Unlike Ernesto, who has always said he'd like to visit his native land so he could see how it has changed, she says she has no desire to set foot there again. When asked if she thinks it should be legal for people to buy and sell their organs, Sandra says, "Yes." Like Ernesto, she sees it as a way to make more organs available to more people. When asked if she'd like to tell any stories of her own about her adventures or her kidney transplant, Sandra shakes her head, giggles, and says, "No."

Ernesto explains, "There's a good reason why Sandra is so shy and doesn't like to talk about herself. She grew up in a very dangerous place at a very dangerous time. Everyone knew what was going on in Guatemala back then, but no one talked about it. Why? Because it was dangerous to talk about it. People would band together to protect each other with their silence. If a stranger came to the village and asked about someone we knew, we'd all go *shush*"—and here Ernesto raises his finger to his lips—"and we wouldn't answer. We all kept quiet about each other and about . . . those other things . . . because we knew the situation around us wasn't any good."

Flashing his big, white smile, Ernesto continues, "Remember I talked about going back to Guatemala after my aunt Otilia died? Remember I said Gicela came up to me after the funeral and said she was sorry my aunt had died? Well, how did Gicela know Otilia was my aunt and not my mother? After all, my sister and my brother both thought Otilia was their mother. The answer is simple. Gicela and I grew up at the same time in Aldea. She was much closer in age to me than to Sandra or Edgar. She could remember on her own when I first came to live in the village in 1984, when I was 11 years old. She knew from her personal experience, without ever being told, that I couldn't be Otilia's own son. But people in Aldea never talked about such things."

Finally Ernesto finishes his train of thought: "It was like living in Iraq today. Very dangerous. There were jobs enough, but people couldn't sleep at night. You'd sleep for 2 or 3 hours at a time. But you could never make it through the night. There were just too many noises to keep you awake. Gunshots in the distance. And you could hear the dogs. The soldiers used dogs to search for the people they wanted. The barking of the dogs would keep you up all night."

For those in need of an organ transplant, the dogs never stop barking. Whether it's day or night, you can't escape their howl: Get an organ or die! And while the Free Market Camp battles the Human Rights Camp, people do indeed die. Dr. Igal Kam fights on the front lines to save as many as he can. About a month after I returned from Prague, I visited him in his office at University Hospital, a neat and modest space with no sweeping view of the Rockies, standard-issue furniture, sturdy like the man. It was still more than a year before the hospital would move to its shiny new campus east of town. He was sitting on his little couch.

At the time, if you had looked closely at Dr. Kam, you'd have seen something in person that was not revealed in his official university photo. There he appeared as a smiling, jovial, stout, gray-haired man who looked a bit like Marlon Brando before he became a whale. In person, he seemed sterner, more cordial than jovial, more sturdy than stout. His hair was actually silver, his eyes very sharp, even predatory, and his skin was the weathered tan of the sabra—a native-born Israeli, darkened by the desert sun.

He opened his mouth and his words spilled forth fast and furious, sometimes with a flourish, and with a residual Israeli accent. You heard both sides of him in his voice. There was the friendly, gracious transplant surgeon, but more. There was also an edge to his voice, some brusqueness that served to emphasize his passion and experience.

It is an edge common among Israelis. It comes from hypervigilance. Israel is always at war. Violence is all too common. Igal Kam didn't wait to begin his mandatory service at 18, but rather, with his parents' permission, volunteered for the air force at 17½. He wanted to fly. He became a pilot cadet. Recalling this period, he laughed—the jovial Dr. Kam—waved his hand, and said, "But they kicked me out and I ended up commanding a battery of antiaircraft missiles outside Tel Aviv."

What kind of missiles? "Hawk missiles," he answered.

What wars did he fight in? "Oh," he said casually, "the Six-Day War in 1967 and all the others. Always there are wars in Israel."

Igal Kam served 5-plus years in the air force. When he was 23, he left the service, no longer a youth. He said, "You learn a lot from doing military service. How to grow up. You know people who die. You see what's really important in life."

Why did he choose medicine? "You would not believe it," said Dr. Kam, again waving his hand. He explained that he applied to study economics at Tel Aviv University, but was rejected because of his low high school grades. "It was a big blow," he recalled.

But the same thing had happened to a friend named Moshe Daniel. They each said, "I'll show them I'm worth more than they think," and together they went to the university in Pisa, Italy, for premedical studies. After that, Dr. Kam returned to his native Haifa for his "clinical" medical education at the Technion–Israel Institute of Technology in Technion City. Moshe Daniel stayed in Italy for his medical degree and returned to Israel to become an orthopedic surgeon who was later awarded a medal for his service in the reserves. The two have remained friends over the years. "Once you go to medical school," said Dr. Kam, "it changes completely your perspective. It's hard to measure the impact it has on you at first."

After his fellowship at the University of Pittsburgh, Dr. Kam returned to Israel and tried to start a liver transplant program there. He was not successful at the time.

He explained that medicine was very political in Israel. And a matter of economics. Many Jews who came to live in Palestine before Independence were communists or socialists. They were thinkers and doers. Israel inherited its ideas about socialized medicine from them. And socialized medicine is always about economics and budgets.

On one side, Dr. Kam expounded, there were the unions that represented the doctors and other health care professionals, and on the other side there were the state hospitals run by the government. There was not, at the time, a strong insurance industry in Israel to subsidize an individual's health care needs, but there was a strong system of private hospitals that had grown in response. When Israel decreased its medical budgets, sophisticated medical procedures like organ transplantation were the first to suffer.

"Some people at Hadassah," said Dr. Kam, meaning the Hadassah Medical Center in Jerusalem, "went ballistic over the idea of starting a transplant program. Especially the doctors who did higher volume but less sophisticated medicine. Already they were fighting for government funds. So they were threatened by it." He tried to preach to them the lessons he had learned during his fellowship at the University of Pittsburgh.

"Because there were no [liver] transplant programs in Israel,

Israelis who could afford it went to the United States for their transplants. They would pay up to $250,000 to do this. If only 2 or 3 cases went abroad each year, that was enough to do 30 cases in Israel. It actually hurt the economy to not have good transplant programs there."

But the system would not budge. Still, despite his political setbacks, Dr. Kam has always loved his work. He reminded me that the first rule for doctors is to do no harm. Then he explained that one of the real challenges with live kidney and liver donations is to be as safe as medically possible with the donor.

"You're taking a healthy person and cutting into them. Is that doing 'no harm'? So there's a risk. So you have to minimize it. But there are so many people who need organs and their need is so desperate. The people who love them won't bypass any opportunity to help, especially if it's a family member."

When the subject of the "transplant outlaw," Zaki Shapira, came up, Dr. Kam—the stern Dr. Kam—frowned and said, "Yeah, I know him well. I've lived with him my whole career. Israel has a very small transplant community. Working in the same field, we couldn't help but cross paths." He paused, shook his silvery head, waved his hand, and continued.

"He's always somewhere . . . in the air. He used to be the head of transplant services at Beilinson Medical Center near Tel Aviv, but these days he's mostly retired. He was investigated, as I'm sure you know, many times. It was in the news."

At first, according to the Israeli media, Dr. Shapira would smuggle Palestinian donors from the West Bank into Israel. He'd get them past the checkpoints, make all the arrangements, broker the organ, and perform the surgery. This was eventually stopped. "I could never accept what he was doing," frowned Dr. Kam, "and I told him so. He insisted he was just trying to help his patients. But after the government stopped him in Tel Aviv, he simply moved his operations to Turkey, Estonia, and Latvia, where he could find all the poor donors he needed. In Estonia, rumors say, he caused a crisis that ended in the resignation of the minister of health."

There was clearly no love lost between the two Israeli surgeons.

Dr. Kam suggested that it was both personal and professional. When he tried to set up a liver transplant program in Israel and needed the support of Dr. Shapira—at the time a legitimate doctor who ran the country's kidney transplant program—there was no support forthcoming. "I needed his goodwill and didn't get it," said Dr. Kam.

And what was worse, Dr. Shapira would not offer available organs that he could not use in his own program to other programs to allow them to grow. So it was a turf war. The politics of Israeli medicine and the economics of its socialized health care system made it professionally impossible for Dr. Kam to start the program he wanted to start.

He recalled a particularly personal story: "A daughter of a friend of mine committed suicide. I went to his house to sit shivah"—the Jewish mourning tradition of visiting the bereaved and saying prayers with them during the 7-day period after the burial—"and my friend said to me, 'Well, at least you got to use her liver, so someone else can live.' And I said to him, 'No, I was never offered her liver. I don't know anything about it.'"

According to Dr. Kam, it was Zaki Shapira who was supposed to have offered him the liver of his friend's daughter. At the time it was a personal blow. But so many years later, Dr. Kam just shrugged philosophically and said, "The environment was simply not ready for it. It was like an amateur program. It still is over there. There are still very few transplants done there, and there are still many people who go abroad to get their transplants. Israel needs rules—new rules, better rules—before it will have the right environment for a first-class transplant program."

And as harsh as his words were for Dr. Shapira as a particular example, they were even harsher for the organ markets in general. Dr. Kam heaped scorn upon organ brokers. He referred to them as "mediators," then stopped himself and said, "Mediators, brokers—whatever. They take such a big percent of what the donor gets. I call them pimps."

He explained how the organ markets would shift from region to region in response to government crackdowns. Most nations agreed that organ trading was criminal. The issue was one of enforcement. At the time, 13 months after my transplant, according to Dr. Kam, the epicenter was shifting again, this time to Central America.

"Go ahead, go to Medellín [Colombia]," he said, "and ask yourself: Why don't the locals get any organs for transplants? How do the mediators get their donors?"

Today, as we have seen, the epicenter is shifting yet again, from Colombia and China to Pakistan and the Philippines. For Dr. Kam, the ethical issues have been even more important than the safety issues. With kidneys and livers, he explained, if the organ is not diseased, then most doctors think they can use it. So what was the problem?

"The problem," said Dr. Kam, "is the potential for organ marketing. It goes against donation. You see, money is stronger than the desire to donate. Marketing will kill donation."

Later, when he said he'd like to "kill the brokering," I noted that he had specified the activity, not the people, but I wondered still at the passion of the man with the eyes that had guided Hawk missiles. Then he spoke as the innovator, the problem solver, the man educated at the Technion. He explained that you have to start by looking at the need and the availability. There are plenty of organs out there. People die. What, then, is the solution?

Here Dr. Kam made a careful distinction between two competing systems that often are confused with each other: What he called marketing schemes, where private parties, generally recipients or their families, pay money to donors or their families, versus proposed compensation schemes, where, pursuant to properly enacted laws, the government would offer incentives to donors or their families. Such incentives could include better health insurance, tax credits, or direct payments: "Whatever the legislature decides."

Dr. Kam was opposed to marketing schemes, but openly favored compensation. "Yes, I'm for it. Today, most deceased donors are already poor people. They're the ones that die from gunshot wounds and accidents. Who gives authority? Who says families that donate their organs should get nothing?" He pointed out everyone else in the chain of supply and demand—hospitals, doctors, nurses, ambulance drivers—all get paid.

Why shouldn't the families of organ donors?

Dr. Kam believed that compensating them would substantially increase the pool of organ donors. All we need is for the government to step in and help. He made it sound, in fact, like exploitation when we don't provide compensation for organ donation. He said, "Look at the value of a single deceased donor. I mean the financial value. It could be a million dollars. One deceased donor can provide a liver, a heart, a pancreas, bowel segments, two kidneys, two lungs, two corneas, bones, and skin."

Dr. Kam was passionate about the solution he was suggesting. He was even more animated than when he talked about the "organ outlaw." He said, "Families have to change their perspectives on donation. And the government must step in, especially when the so-called free market is knocking on the door."

He took a deep breath and slowed down to admit that he did not have all the details. He could not answer specific questions about the mechanics of a compensation system. He protested, "I'm just the doctor, the guy with the ideas. It's up to the policy makers and lawmakers to figure out the details. But it is clear—there are studies that have shown—that compensation would provide more organs. And offering real value through a system run by the government avoids the exploitation of the market system."

Critics from the Free Market Camp might snort, pointing to Dr. Kam's heritage, and suggest that you can take the man out of the socialized system, but you can't take the socialized system out of the man. And critics from the Human Rights Camp might sneer and insist that payment is payment is payment: The system described by Dr. Kam would still exploit the poor. But he is no champion of Israel's system. He was not speaking about socialism. And he argued that he was the one who was avoiding exploitation.

I thought, *Maybe he is on to something.* There were, after all, the ideologues. Then there were the experienced, hardheaded pragmatists looking for solutions to a daunting social and medical problem. Dr. Kam argued, "Why turn to brokers—mediators, pimps—when the solution is right before you? We have enough potential donors to satisfy our needs. We need to give them more incentives to donate. Compensation gives them incentives. Payment from a market system exploits them."

When he did turn to specifics—my case in particular—Dr. Kam was vehement: "There is no way to convince me it would have been better for you to go to Turkey."

But Dr. Kam did not take the opportunity to further slam Dr. Shapira. Instead, he said, "Why go there? You didn't know the donor or the doctors. You'd get your kidney, then 3 days later—poof!—they'd be gone. If you'd had any problems, you would have had to go somewhere else for care. And complications can lead to real problems after transplants. When you don't have the same doctors who did the surgery available afterward, the risks are so much greater. The results can be disastrous."

No wonder Dr. Kam so adamantly opposed the idea that I might go to Turkey to buy that supposedly Israeli kidney from Zaki Shapira. The ethical, safety, and other reasons all came into play for Dr. Kam. For him, there was only one option.

There in his office, he said to me the same thing he had said many times before: "You had a perfect match with your son. That's very unusual, you know. Usually you only find a perfect match with siblings. In your case, it was simply lack of knowledge that was driving you away."

So the Band-Aid approach does not work, presumed consent is not the answer, and the United States simply is not prepared to adopt a true free market system in organs. Would Dr. Kam's suggestion that we adopt a compensated donation system work in a meaningful way? Could we create such a system that was consistent with our legal values, our economic limitations, and our political will?

In fact, since the time when Dr. Kam first explained to me the benefits of compensated donation, important voices have joined him in offering the same solution. Economists Gary S. Becker from the University of Chicago and Julio Jorge Elías of the State University of New York at Buffalo have argued that "monetary incentives could increase the supply of organs for transplant sufficiently to eliminate even the large queues in the organ market. And it would do this without increasing the total cost of transplant surgery by a large percent."[1] Becker and Elías cover a lot of the same ground we've seen before: The very low risk of a live donor dying as a result of a kidney transplant ("We . . . estimate that the risk of death . . . is 0.1 percent"[2]), the inapplicability of free market data from emerging countries like India and Iran ("the experience in these two low-income nations is hardly comparable to what would happen in the United States"[3]), the inability of "presumed consent" to close the gap between supply and demand.

These economists are, in fact, particularly critical of presumed consent systems—also known as opt-out arrangements. They say, "We believe that presumed consent is a dangerous principle, and that in the absence of clear directive from the decedent, heirs should control the remains of loved ones. . . . [T]he 'presumed consent' organ procurement approach will not eliminate the long queues for transplants. [One study] indicates that presumed consent systems may reduce rather than raise the number of organs donated."[4]

But Becker and Elías go further in their elaborate use of tables, graphs, models, and analysis that builds upon the existing "value of life literature." They compare compensated donation with America's volunteer army, for example, and conclude that the former would be no more troublesome than the latter is.[5] What the economists do not address is where the money for compensated donation would come from. If it comes from those in need of the organs themselves, then it is really no different than a free market system.

If, however, the money does not come from those in need of the organs, then who foots the bill? Enter Arthur Matas, MD, from the University of Minnesota. His analysis, "A Gift of Life Deserves Compensation," prepared for the Cato Institute, addresses this and many of the other issues I encountered during my trip through the transplant maze.[6] He starts with a different tack, however: "Treatment for end-stage renal . . . disease . . . is the only government-funded health care in the United States that has no financial need- or age-based criteria." And he concludes with a very different response: "The best way to increase the supply of kidneys without drastically changing the existing allocation system is to legalize a regulated system of compensation for living kidney donors."[7]

In between, Dr. Matas provides the sort of specifics that Dr. Kam was unable to provide when I first spoke with him about compensated donation. Yes, he covers ground that's grown familiar. He observes, for example, that paired exchanges, like those authorized by the recent amendments to NOTA, "only provide a relatively small number of new donors."[8] Then, one by one, he debunks all the myths: "Policymakers confuse a [compensated donation] system with what happens when there is a black market in organs. . . . No potential compensated donor can be coerced by the opportunity to be compensated. . . . The system advocated here is constructed to prevent exploitation."[9]

Ultimately, he says, "At the end of the day, one must cut through all the passion and rhetoric and ask this very simple question: What is the better option—establishing a system of compensation (even if doing so might not be easy) or maintaining the status quo (under which transplant candidates are suffering and dying on dialysis)?"[10]

His choice is clear. But what are the specifics that make Dr. Matas's proposal meaningfully different? Here is how his system would work.[11]

The procedural framework would be virtually identical to the system currently used to evaluate altruistic living donor organs, but the allocation system would be the one currently used for altruistic deceased donor organs. The deceased donor model . . . is appropriate because there currently is no official allocation system in place for living organ donations. At this point almost all living donor organ donations are directed donations to family or friends. Thus, by combining current existing models for living and deceased organ procurement and allocation, a system can be developed that provides the following: a predefined algorithm, such as the one used by UNOS, to assure that everyone on the waiting list has the same opportunity to undergo a transplant, full evaluation of potential donors, informed consent, careful oversight, long-term follow-up, and treatment of donors with dignity. . . . The added element proposed here is a fixed payment to donors by the government or a government-approved agency (hereafter I will use the term compensated donation). Existing prohibitions on private sales would remain in place.

Compensation for donors could take many forms. Options include a fixed payment, long-term health insurance, college tuition, tax deductions, or some combination of these alternatives or other equally valuable forms of compensation. . . . A menu of options would provide each donor with something that has personal value. For example, health insurance may be of value to those who do not have work-related health insurance but not to others. A tax break may be of value to some, direct compensation to others. Under the system advocated here, no other commercialization would be allowed. All legal allocation of organs and payment for organs would take place through the government or a government-determined contractor. Currently existing prohibitions on private brokers and contact between the donor and recipient would remain in place.

Wow! Let's take a closer look at this. It looks like the Iranian system adapted to our modern capitalist, democratic context. It uses several elements we have seen before, like the tax breaks proposed in Michigan and the economic incentives for donors that are championed by the Free Market Camp. But it also has protections for donors that do not exist in America today, so it should make the Human Rights Camp happy. It avoids the legal problems with presumed consent, it avoids the exploitation characteristic of the black markets, and it provides a range of choices for donors to choose from. I am particularly attracted to the idea of giving living donors long-term care and health insurance.

And compensated donation is less disruptive to the existing system than any other serious option. Even before the recent amendments to NOTA, federal law excluded some types of compensation from the idea of valuable consideration: "Reasonable payments associated with the removal, transportation, implantation, processing, preservation, quality control, and storage of a human organ or the expenses of travel, housing, and lost wages incurred by the donor of a human organ in connection with the donation."[12] This was the language that permitted Rob Smitty to receive some payment in connection with the donation of his kidney to Bob Hickey in that first match made by a commercial Internet Web site. It is what allows Pennsylvania, Delaware, and Michigan to experiment by establishing trust fund payments in limited amounts for donors' actual expenses.

I am convinced that compensated donation along the lines proposed by Dr. Kam and Dr. Matas is doable economically, politically, and legally. It would provide a major part of the solution to the crisis in our organ transplant policy. I base this opinion on my experiences, since my own transplant, with doctors, academics, legislators, and fellow lawyers; on my activities in promoting organ transplant reform; and on common sense.

Another big part of the solution to our organ transplant crisis lies in stimulating rather than repressing stem cell research. Already today, before we're able to clone actual organs, we've seen breakthroughs that could revolutionize transplant medicine. It is time for America to stop holding back its scientists with political nonsense. Fortunately, since becoming president, Barack Obama appears to be making good on his promise to reinstate science to its critical role in determining sound government policy. He realizes that it is long past time for us to catch up to the rest of the world when it comes to the realities of the brave new frontiers of science and medicine.

At the same time that Dr. Kam was telling me about compensated donation, roughly 13 months after my surgery, stem cell research was capturing the news. What exactly are these things we call stem cells? They have been called the body's basic building blocks and hailed as medicine's new frontier. They are cells that are undifferentiated—they do not have a specific bodily function—and self-replicating—they can divide and replicate repeatedly.[13]

They are the types of cells found in human embryos.

As Dr. Larry Chan explained, stem cells hold the key to the future of organ transplants. They are already being used to assist traditional transplants by bolstering the recipient's immune system; it is hoped that they will soon be used to grow new organ tissue, and that someday they could be used as "bioreactors" that merge tissues with machines.

And most important, someday they will be used to grow entirely new organs.

Research into artificial organs is being actively pursued by universities and institutions around the world, including McGill University's Artificial Cells and Organs Research Center[14] in Montreal and the McGowan Institute for Regenerative Medicine at the University of Pittsburgh, where Dr. Kam first specialized in kidney and liver transplants.[15] Today, he is concerned that stem cell research and artificial organs could be "more about future dreams than the solutions we need now." But that's not why it is controversial.

Stem cell research is controversial in America because some people believe it destroys human embryos and therefore human beings. Many others disagree. The issue is political and emotional and the stakes are exceedingly high.

After President George W. Bush limited stem cell research severely during his first term, voters in California approved a $3 billion bond initiative to fund stem cell research in their state over the next 10 years. Other states—including Illinois, Connecticut, Indiana, Maryland, Massachusetts, New Jersey, New York, Ohio, Virginia, and Wisconsin—have joined the movement toward state funding of stem cell research.[16]

Plainly, stem cell research is both highly political and highly economic in nature. That is why it was front-page news when the US

House of Representatives, led by Republican Mike Castle of Delaware and Democrat Diana DeGette of Colorado, in May 2005, by a vote of 238–194, passed the Stem Cell Research Enhancement Act.[17] It was a modest effort that would have granted federally funded researchers access to new stem cell lines if the embryos used to derive the stem cells were originally created for fertility treatment purposes and were in excess of clinical need, if the people donating the embryos gave written permission for their use, and if the embryos would otherwise be discarded by the fertility clinic. Later, after the Senate also passed this legislation, President Bush exercised his very first veto to kill it.[18] His veto set America back years in therapeutic stem cell research.

Meanwhile, in South Korea, according to the *New York Times*, "biomedical researchers reported that they had developed an efficient method for obtaining human stem cells from embryos produced through cloning."[19] But the South Korean scientists did not get their cloned embryos by fertilizing human eggs. Rather, they removed the genetic material from donated eggs and replaced it with genetic material from cells of patients. In fact, the scientists who had achieved this breakthrough had been very careful not to even use the word "clone" to describe what they did.[20]

Instead, the scientists called it "somatic cell nuclear transfer" that produced "human nuclear transfer blastocysts" from which they could extract "hESC"—meaning human embryonic stem cells. The apparent euphemizing in the use of language was partially explained by the headline, "Name Games and the Science of Life," which demonstrated how proponents on both sides "manipulate language" in the debates over stem cell research.

Dr. Woo Suk Hwang, who led the South Korean team, insisted, "I never destroy any life during my process. . . . We use only a vacant egg, with no genetic materials. . . . On the one hand, you have 15 micrometers of skin cells, on the other a patient who has suffered from an incurable disease. Maybe this 15 micrometers of skin cells can relieve and save the life of a human being next to me, someone who has suffered for 50 years or must suffer for 50 years. Of the two, which do you think is ethically reasonable to save?"[21]

The problem was that Dr. Hwang was a fraud. His report was totally discredited.[22] The debate shifted to the enforcement of proper scientific standards when evaluating claims of major medical advances. The shift showed just how globalized science had become, implicating deep divisions in politics, economics, and law.

Still, despite President Bush's veto of the Stem Cell Research Enhancement Act and setbacks like the fraud perpetrated by the South Korean scientists, polls consistently show that Americans overwhelmingly support stem cell research.[23] One poll demonstrated that the more accurate information people are given about stem cell research, the more they approve of it. And despite the restrictions placed upon it by the Bush administration, the scientific community has responded with an avalanche of stunning medical advances. What follow are just a few of the most important advances in stem cell research and transplant medicine of the past few years.

Growing Stem Cells from Skin Cells

In June 2007, the *New York Times* reported on a "surprising advance that could sidestep the ethical debates surrounding stem cell biology."[24] The advance was an easy technique for reprogramming the skin cells of a mouse to return to their embryonic state. Assuming that this technique could be adapted to humans, scientists could use a patient's skin cells to generate new heart, liver, or kidney cells that would be transplantable and would not be rejected by the patient's immune system. Before, the only way to convert adult cells to their embryonic state had been by nuclear transfer, inserting the nucleus of an adult cell into an egg whose nucleus had been removed. That procedure, known as therapeutic cloning, has not yet been successful in humans.

With the new technique, developed by Shinya Yamanaka, MD, of Kyoto University in Japan, four genes inserted into a single skin cell reprogram the cell to take its embryonic state. The technique is easier to perform than nuclear transfer and doesn't use human eggs, so it shouldn't pose the ethical problems some see with the use of embryonic stem cells. David Scadden, MD, a stem cell biologist at Harvard Medical School, said the new technique "is truly extraordinary and frankly something most assumed would take a decade to work out."

Perhaps most importantly, the new technique "raises no serious moral problem, because it creates embryoniclike stem cells without creating, harming or destroying human lives at any stage," said Richard Doerflinger, spokesman for the United States Conference of Catholic Bishops on stem cell issues.

Scientists Create a Beating Heart in the Lab

In January 2008, researchers at the University of Minnesota announced that they had created a beating heart in the laboratory.[25] The scientists stripped the existing cells from a dead heart so that only the protein "skeleton" remained, the part that basically gives shape to the heart. Then the structure was "seeded with live 'progenitor' cells, which multiplied and grew back over it, eventually linking together in a new organ." Doris Taylor, PhD, the principal researcher on the project, said, "The idea would be to develop transplantable blood vessels or whole organs that are made from your own cells." The advantage, of course, would be that organs built in this manner would use stem cells taken from the patient's own body, so its immune system would not reject them. Say good-bye to immunosuppressants!

"It opens a door to the notion that you can make any organ—

kidney, liver or pancreas," said Dr. Taylor. "You name it and we hope we can make it."

Consider the implications: The process used powerful chemicals to strip those dead cells from the dead heart and the progenitor cells that were used to seed the skeleton were taken from the hearts of newborn animals. Four days after seeding, the cells could be seen contracting, and after 8 days the heart itself started contracting.

"We took nature's building blocks to build a new organ," declared coresearcher Harald Ott. "When we saw the first contractions, we were speechless."

"This is proof of concept," Taylor added. "Going forward, our goal is to use a patient's stem cells to build a new heart."

No More Immunosuppressants

Also in January 2008, three reports in the *New England Journal of Medicine* gave new hope to transplant recipients: Someday soon they could be free of their immunosuppressant drugs.[26] The treatment involved weakening a kidney recipient's immune system with intravenous drugs several days before the transplant, then giving the recipient an infusion of bone marrow from the donor to create a new immune system. Stem cells from the marrow would "trick" the immune system into thinking the new organ had come from the recipient himself. In one experiment, four of five kidney recipients were entirely off immunosuppressant drugs up to 5 years later.

"The ability to achieve tolerance in what's called stable chimerism [when donor cells are present in the recipient] in patients has been postulated since the 1960s," said W. Roy Smythe, MD, from Texas A&M's medical school. "It's really been a 'gee whiz' thing for the last 30 years [but] this is proof of principle in human beings, which is a big deal."

Elimination of antirejection drugs in the near future was something that really got my attention. I am, after all, a kidney recipient, and for most recipients, it's a lifelong commitment to drugs. Imagine: no prednisone, no Coumadin, no awful side effects—hair growth, bloating, tremors, diabetes, an even greater risk of cancer.

No sooner did one of our friends call attention to this advance, however, than I could see the old anger flare in Cindy's eyes: "If you think for 1 minute you're going back to Gregg for a bone marrow transplant, you're crazy!"

Maybe she is right. I have already drunk from that well of life. But there is one more transplant advance that shows without question that the future is now.

Remember that John Woo movie *Face/Off* with John Travolta and Nicolas Cage? Bad guy Cage swaps faces with good guy Travolta using the latest in face transplant technology. All hell breaks loose. Bad guy seduces good guy's wife. Lots of martial arts and bullets flying in operatic slow motion. Pure science fiction, right? Wrong!

"Woman Has First Face Transplant"

That was the headline on the BBC News Web site on November 30, 2005.[27] The 38-year-old French patient was severely disfigured. She had lost her nose, lips, and chin after her pet Labrador chewed her face while she was passed out from an overdose of sleeping pills. She had been unable to speak or eat properly ever since. The surgery was performed only after she received extensive counseling to ensure that she understood the medical risks—she would have to take powerful immunosuppressant drugs for the rest of her life—and the emotional risks: She would likely not look like she had before.

The patient went ahead with the surgery, receiving not only a partial face transplant from a 46-year-old brain-dead woman, but also an injection of the donor's bone marrow cells. The surgery was pronounced a success. Two years later, researchers in Cincinnati and Louisville reported the immunosuppressive risks associated with facial transplants were lower than expected, and on the 2nd anniversary of the transplant, the lead surgeon, Jean-Michel Dubernard, MD, proclaimed, "She's perfect."[28] Which meant she could smile and eat much better, despite experiencing kidney failure and two episodes in which her body's immune system had tried to reject her new face.

Still, in March 2008, the Facial Surgery Research Foundation in London hosted a public debate on facial transplantation, tissue engineering, and the impact on identity.[29] Among the topics: growing faces in the laboratory and tissue for faces inside the hospitable environment of the patient's own body.

By then, however, doctors in France and China had performed the second and third partial face transplants. And in December 2008, doctors at the Cleveland Clinic performed the first face transplant in the United States and the first near-total face transplant in the world.[30] These operations, though still experimental, have raised ethical concerns that center on the face as a marker of identity. But such concerns seem, to me, to be easily outweighed by medicine's ability to restore a living face that is horribly disfigured.

I only wish I could have been there to watch the 23-hour operation. I can't understand the opposition in America to stem cell research. The arguments against it seem so abstract to me: Human life begins at conception and absolutely nothing can be done to that life once it is conceived. Even if it's only a handful of self-replicating cells? And the arguments in favor of it seem so compelling, not just to me, but to the 65 to 75 percent of Americans who support increased stem cell research.

We commonly allow women to sell their eggs to fertility clinics.[31] Does it really make sense, from the standpoint of public policy, to allow eggs to be bought and sold to make babies while objecting to therapeutic stem cell research in the same breath? Is it moral to create lives but not to save lives by curing disease? How can we allow human organs to be bought and sold for research and teaching purposes, but not for transplant purposes?

I believe that a "culture of life" should honor actual lives in being as much as—if not more than—those with the potential to become such. Besides, the genie of technology is out of the bottle. It can never be pushed back in.

In the short term, compensated donation holds the most promise among the options for solving our crisis in organ transplant policy in America. In the long term, stem cell research will yield even more stunning advances in transplant medicine. Together, this two-pronged attack can shrink or eliminate our organ waiting lists.

And save many lives.

CHAPTER THIRTEEN

A NEW LIFE AND NEW PURPOSE

It was only after I survived my second battle with kidney disease that I learned of a letter in my medical file, written to my childhood doctors in Denver by the specialists at the Mayo Clinic. It was dated February 12, 1946. I have memorized one sentence: "We certainly cannot be any more optimistic than you have been over the future of this boy."

Reading that letter for the first time, I finally understood what my mother meant when she used to tell me, "There was a reason you were allowed to live."

So I have set up the American Transplant Foundation[1] to improve the system.

That is the purpose my mother had foreseen for me.

My goal is to eliminate our nation's tragic shortage of transplant organs. Through my nonprofit foundation, I intend to help other families understand and deal with the challenges faced by transplant patients and their loved ones. We are helping to fund a professor's chair in transplant medicine at the new University of Colorado Health Sciences Center. We have already secured changes to Colorado's income tax forms to make it easier to designate oneself as an organ donor. Crosby, Stills and Nash performed a benefit concert for us in the summer of 2008. David Crosby, of course, had a liver transplant in 1994. I have also joined the board of the Donor Alliance Council,[2] the organ procurement organization that obtains and distributes transplant organs in the region that includes Colorado.

But there is so much more to do.

Transplants are transformative. They save lives and they change lives. Since I got my new kidney, I have become a poster boy for organ transplantation. I have added to my hectic schedule of law practice, charitable work, and political activity a new dimension: spokesman for improving America's organ transplant system. Now, of course, I am not alone in pursuing this goal, but I am well suited to the task.

When the University of Colorado celebrated its 1,000th liver transplant, I attended a big dinner to mark the occasion. There I ran into Chris Klug, the famous Olympic snowboard medalist. He had suffered from a rare degenerative bile duct condition, and Dr. Kam gave him a liver transplant at University Hospital in 2000. Some time before the dinner, he and I were supposed to be interviewed together by Fox News. Chris had already published his book, *To the Edge and Back: My Story from Organ Transplant Survivor to Olympic Snowboarder*. So he had been around the track as one of the celebrities who were organ transplant poster boys.

Unfortunately, he did not show up for the Fox News interview, and I was forced to go it alone. So later, when I ran into him at the University of Colorado dinner, I asked, "Dude, why didn't you come to the interview?"

Now, Chris didn't really talk that way—calling everybody "dude"—but I found myself talking that way around him to tease him. He answered in the same teasing manner: "Dude, I had other things I had to do. It had just snowed, you see, and I'm a boarder. That's what I do. I board. I'm sorry, but I just couldn't make it that day."

Since Chris had done more than his share of organ donor awareness work, I could hardly fault him for missing yet another interview about it. But I do not have his excuse. It is a critical part of my job—my role in both my personal and professional lives—to do fundraising and other things for charitable organizations.

That is what I do: raise money, speak out, promote causes, pursue missions.

And when it comes to organ transplants, I am a man on a mission. I want my journey through the transplant maze to help guide others on their journeys. For despite all the trials, tribulations, and tough decisions we faced, Gregg's donation to me and Ernesto's to his sister are both great success stories.

We have all recovered from our surgeries. We are all leading normal lives. For me, that means long hours of work—for clients, charities, politicians, and political causes—and time with my family and friends whenever I'm not attending some big-deal function or flying somewhere. For Ernesto, it means raising his two kids, continuing to build his business, and staying afloat in tough economic times. Seldom does he even think about his transplant experience.

The same is not true for everyone. Not all transplant journeys cross waters as smooth as those we sailed. Recall that fashion guru Steven Cojocaru, one of my growing circle of "transplant friends," found himself back in the hospital 6 months after his transplant. The kidney he had received had become infected and had to be removed. His mother stepped forward and donated one of her kidneys to him. He had a second transplant and has since recovered, published his own transplant memoir, and returned to the red carpet.

A week or so after Cojo went back to the hospital to receive his mother's kidney, Fox News came to my house to shoot some footage of Gregg and me. Shaul Turner, a local TV personality and the recent recipient of the Donor Awareness Council's Excellence in Journalism Award, came out with her cameraman and an intern.

Then we started a game of HORSE around the basketball hoop in the driveway. It was midafternoon and the temperature was in the mid-90s, and since there was more sweating than bantering, the little microphones they'd put on us couldn't have been getting much more than our heavy breathing.

Gregg shot and missed, then I shot and missed. We frowned. It got competitive. He hit his shot, then I hit mine and, *swish* for *swish*, we both hit.

Shaul asked her cameraman, "Did you get that?"

He nodded and said, "Yep."

"Then let's wrap it here," she said, "and move around back."

We all walked around to the little putting green I have behind my home. I had worked up a sweat shooting those hoops and was feeling good. Gregg and I took turns putting from about 30 feet from the pin. I was the first to sink one, but he matched me fairly soon after that, and then we each sank another for the cameraman.

By then we were both feeling hot from the blazing summer sun, so we went over to some chairs we had under the trees and sat in the shade while Shaul asked us follow-up questions. Like the reporter from the *Denver Post*, she had interviewed us before.

Gregg and I each held our putters. I also had my tennis racket on my lap, ready for the next activity. Gregg was answering a question: "I feel so lucky that I was such a good match, that my father could be saved. I just needed to be there for him. You know how he uses his connections in such a positive manner? You know, there's nothing in the world he wouldn't do for anyone in the world." I felt so proud of him for saying that.

Then Shaul took the mike from Gregg and we threaded it under my shirt. And I was answering a question: "I have such a good life. I'm so thankful for my loving son and for the opportunity to share my time with my kids, my new granddaughter, my wife, and friends." I never get tired of saying those things.

Next, I led everyone past the pool to the tennis court.

I turned my baseball cap around and hit some balls with Gregg.

By then it was *really* hot and we were *really* sweating. Still, even after Shaul said, "That's all we need for now," and the cameraman turned off his Canon, we kept hitting those balls. We were hitting them hard by then. It felt so good. Gregg and I had remained as naturally competitive as we had always been.

When we finally got tired and came off the court, someone asked, "After all that exertion, how do you feel?" This is a question I get asked a lot since my transplant.

I smiled and told the truth: "I feel fine."

Rumor has it that Zaki Shapira moved his operations to the Philippines soon after his release from that Turkish jail. These sorts of rumors are pretty hard to verify, however. What's clear is that the organ markets have continued to grow, with or without him.

Will they keep growing? Some say the economics of globalization are in retreat. Capitalism has stalled. They point to the excesses of the International Monetary Fund and the World Bank. They point to the many failures of the World Trade Organization. They point to the resurgence of socialism in Latin America. But I don't buy it. Just like Thomas Friedman says, globalization is "inexorable." The Internet has flattened our world and plugged everyone into a capitalist and democratic environment. China has adopted major market reforms. Even Cuba is emerging from communism.

Some also say the politics of democracy are in retreat. They point to the troubling growth of the "predatory state."[3] They point to America's overemphasis on holding elections in troubled nations without building the institutions that could make those elections fair and legitimate. They point to the alarming growth of armed militias all over the world—just look at Hezbollah in Lebanon, the

Taliban in Afghanistan, Hamas in the Palestinian territories, the Janjaweed in Darfur, even Blackwater in America—and argue that sovereignty is facing its biggest challenge yet. But the nation-state isn't going away. Multinational corporations and transsovereign organizations like the United Nations and World Trade Organization are still built upon a base of sovereignty. The European Union's rejection of a single constitution shows that Western sensibilities are not ready to relinquish the comforts of nationalism.

Some even argue that the rule of law has reached its limits in the new millennium. They say it is men who rule the country, not the letter of the law. Some point to the US Supreme Court's willingness to ignore its own precedents in awarding the presidency to George W. Bush in 2000. Some point to the hypocrisies of the Abu Ghraib and Guantánamo Bay prisons. But I say we still operate a freer country than anyone else in the world. And during the presidency of Barack Obama—formerly a professor of constitutional law—we should expect renewed protection of civil rights and liberties. More and more emerging nations are adopting modern commercial codes, labor laws, environmental laws, intellectual property laws, and human rights laws—though their main reason for doing so often lies in their desire to do business with us.

Again we see the intersections of globalization with sovereignty and law.

No, I do not believe the forces of economics, politics, and law have slowed down. The conditions that created the environment for the growth of capitalist markets in transplant organs persist. But America is not an emerging Third World country. Solutions are available to us that are not available to others.

Compensated donation and expanded stem cell research hold the keys to eliminating the organ waiting lists in America. The American dream should include the dream of universal health care that offers organ transplants to all who need them.

As Gregg and I competed on the golf links at Castle Pines a few days after our interview with Fox News, Ernesto was driving his daughter, Galilea; his wife, Gicela; his brother, Edgar; and his four cousins to California for a few days of family vacation at the beach. This was before the birth of Ernesto's son.

They stopped in Las Vegas, but stayed there for only a few hours—"Gee, it was awfully hot there," says Ernesto—before driving 4 more hours to another cousin's home in Santa Monica, California. Gali, for once, had not insisted on bringing along her used Toshiba laptop. She had set her sights on bigger prey: Disneyland!

The following weekend Ernesto proudly showed his photos from the trip at the small reunion that finally brought together the Farber, Sullivan, and Delaroca families. He showed his pictures slowly, proudly, one by one, so we could savor each moment, more of the American dream come true: There's little Gali hugging Mickey Mouse. There's Ernesto wearing a Goofy hat. Then a Nemo hat. Smiling with those dazzling white teeth for the camera, soaking up the moment.

Ernesto was no longer an immigrant peasant from Guatemala. Like me, he too had changed. His landscaping business was taking off and the reunion was being held as much to celebrate the new American entrepreneur as the transplant poster boy. He had not been able to fly all eight members of his extended family to California, but he had been able to afford to rent a big van and take some time off and drive them there.

The reunion took place 16 months after our transplant surgeries. It was in early August 2005. The first to arrive was Lynne, stepping from her bronze Mercedes, green bracelet—"*Done Vida*"—dangling from her wrist. Next, Ernesto came in his purple Toyota pickup truck with Gicela, Gali, and a nephew Gali's age named Harrison. Sandra could not get time off from her job at Wendy's, so she had to miss the reunion. That is why I still have never met her. Next,

I arrived in my black Mercedes; Jim in his black Porsche Cayenne; and finally, Gregg with Cindy and his daughter, Andie, who at the time was 6 months old.

Over fresh bagels and lox, rocket salad with beef tenderloin, potato casserole brought by Lynne, and homemade quiche, two kidney donors and one recipient gathered with their families and friends to honor the day, 16 months before, when their paths had crossed at University Hospital in Denver, where they had shared the same surgeon and the same waiting rooms: indeed, the same transplant experience.

A lot of attention was focused on Andie, my new granddaughter. She was not fussy in the slightest. She spent her time looking painfully cute and sucking on her pink pacifier. Cindy just could not get enough. A grandmother for the first time, she grinned every minute Andie was in her clutches, except for the second or two when she realized Andie was peeing in her lap. Even then, several of the gathered remarked that they hadn't seen Cindy so happy in months.

Meanwhile, Gicela, who grew up in the Guatemalan village of Aldea and still spoke little English, spent most of her time chasing Gali and Harrison as they ran around outside in the August heat. Everything seemed so normal. We all knew we were there "because of the transplants," but at first no one talked about it. We just chatted.

The night before, Cindy, Jim, Lynne, and I had seen a new summer action movie, *The Island*. Lynne had walked out soon after the beginning. At the reunion, she explained, "It was all so obvious. Right away you know what's going to happen. There is no island. These people—the hero and the heroine—are clones and they've been created so the rich people from whom they've been cloned can use their organs for transplant purposes. Then they escape and there's a big chase and lots of explosions."

Surprisingly, even with that opportunity to relate the movie to

The Search for Solutions

208

our experiences, there wasn't much other discussion about transplants at the reunion. Everyone was just catching up and making small talk. At one point, I was wearing a baseball cap backwards and looking as goofy as Ernesto in his Goofy hat at Disneyland. I held Andie aloft and talked some baby talk to her. Someone finally leaned over and whispered to Ernesto, "You know, if it hadn't been for that transplant, Steve wouldn't be here now, holding his grandchild like that."

Ernesto only smiled his big, white smile, shook his head, and said, "Whoa!"

Later, when he and I were sitting close to each other at the table, I asked him, "How is Sandra doing?"

Ernesto answered, "Fine, just fine."

"How long," I asked, "was she on the waiting list?"

He answered, "Over 2½ years."

"So she had to walk to her dialysis for all of those 2½ years?"

"That's right," said Ernesto, "until I gave her my kidney."

Even after that exchange, talk about transplants came only sporadically, buried beneath the chitchat and casual banter that flowed more freely. Still, every time I sat near Ernesto, I started thinking about the similarities between him and my son Gregg. They are almost exactly the same age. They are both family men who are more interested in their young daughters than any talk about kidney transplants or heroism. Neither of them ever sought the limelight. In fact, this modest reunion was one of the exceedingly few times they voluntarily appeared to celebrate their transplant experiences— and this was a tight-knit gathering limited to family and close friends. Yet both Ernesto and Gregg had transcended the fears that naturally come with any decision to donate a live organ, and each had saved the life of a loved one without asking for anything in return.

They were the two who had donated. They were the givers.

I had thought a lot about the contrasts between the Delaroca family and my own, the poor and the rich, the peasant and the power broker. But here, indeed, was the one thing that truly united us all: the love of two selfless people who gave freely of themselves.

Finally, the gathering drew to a close. Near the end, someone asked Ernesto whether he had thought about the transplant at all during his recent vacation in California. It was expected that he would say no, for that would signal a true healing, a turning away from concerns of life and death to concerns of family, business, and fulfilling the American dream. Those were, after all, the reasons Ernesto had brought his family from Guatemala to begin with. Instead, he surprised everyone and said, "Yes, I did think about it while we were gone."

"Really?" asked someone. "What did you think?"

"I thought, Now I can relax. Even though Sandra wasn't with us"—she hadn't been able to get off work to go to California, just as she wasn't able to get off work to attend the reunion—"I knew she'd be okay. Ever since the transplant, she's done so well."

Ernesto paused. A flash of something, some memory perhaps, crossed his eyes, turning them inward. He blinked. Was it the beach at Santa Monica? Or Disneyland? Or was it Gali telling him she loved him before they wheeled him to the operating room? Could it have been his parents being dragged off into the night, never to be seen again? Today, Ernesto does not recall.

But he turned back to the gathering and finished his thought: "I knew everything would be okay."

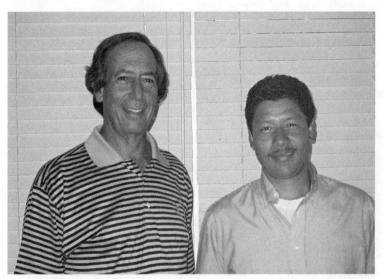

From left: Steve and Ernesto, August 2005

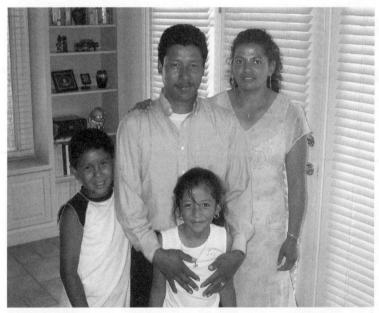

Clockwise from top center: Ernesto with his wife, Gicela; daughter, Galilea; and nephew, Harrison, August 2005

A New Life and New Purpose

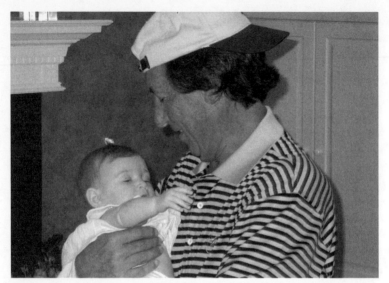

Steve with his granddaughter, Andie

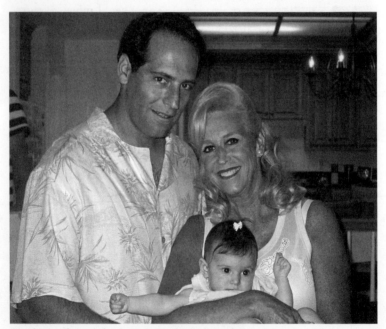

Clockwise from left: Gregg, Cindy, and Andie

EPILOGUE

In the time since Zaki Shapira's arrest in Turkey, I have thought a lot about it. I'm doing a lot of traveling these days, back and forth from the East Coast, where my sons and granddaughter live, and all over the country on business. The Democrats came to Denver last summer and nominated Barack Obama to run as our first African American president. And he actually won! And I didn't just live to see it. I was able to play a real part in it. I cochaired the host committee and raised more than $50 million for the event. It was exhilarating and draining all at the same time.

And it's true: All those hours spent in the air mean that sometimes I get bored with the latest big-deal contract or *Wall Street Journal* or upcoming conference in Los Angeles. Sometimes, 30-some thousand feet over some place I cannot see, I move all those things aside, clear the tray table, and think about the fact that I could have been arrested along with Zaki Shapira in Turkey. I am happier than ever that I did not avail myself of that opportunity.

The growing global markets for human transplant organs were, for me, an option rightly considered and rightly rejected. Forever I will accept the consequences of accepting Gregg's kidney. I don't think I would be able to say the same if I had purchased my organ from some poor guy in the Middle East.

Ernesto, by the way, has a new baby boy. Ernesto Angel Delaroca was born on May 6, 2007—within a few days of Dr. Zaki Shapira's arrest in Turkey! How our paths have diverged since the time they crossed at University Hospital in Denver on the morning of May 11, 2004.

Little Ernesto Jr. looks a lot like his dad: wavy black hair, dark skin, white teeth, the brightest of eyes. And the dad is looking a little plump, just like the kid. Living the American dream can do that to you, I guess.

The stories of our two families convince me—as I hope they convince you—that our nation needs significant reform in its organ transplant policy. After juggling those pesky forces of economics, politics, and law and considering all those clamorous ethical, religious, and other voices, we must act. And the time to act is now. We have a menu of well-developed options to choose from. Some are so much better than others.

The answer does not, for example, lie in modest efforts like the limited amendments recently made to the National Organ Transplant Act and the Uniform Anatomical Gift Act. Those reforms do not go far enough. The answer does not lie in presumed consent, either. It has proven to be insufficiently efficacious in eliminating the organ waiting lists in all but a few places that have tried it. The answer also does not lie in developing free capitalist markets in human organs. Americans are not ready for that—and neither is the rest of the world.

The answer may well be found in a combination of compensated donation, as described in Chapter Twelve, in the shorter term and more stem cell research in the longer term. And no, I won't repeat all of those depressing statistics. By now they've been stated enough.

The engines of the private plane are droning in my ears. My eyelids close, but I am not falling asleep. With the cabin lights shining through them, my lids look like orange movie screens, curved in two places. Not one like IMAX or three like Cinerama. But two: my own private viewing screen.

And on them flashes not *Citizen Kane* or even *Midnight Express.* On them flashes my imaginary cinematic version of the arrest of Zaki Shapira in 2007 in Turkey—with my arrest following close behind. He is led to the police van in his wrinkled green scrubs and his little purple knit cap. I am vaguely aware that the purple knit cap is a detail I have supplied. Next I am wheeled from the little clinic hidden on the Asian side of Istanbul, strapped to a gurney and helpless, keenly aware that something has gone profoundly wrong, but still too drowsy from the anesthesia to do anything about it.

My reflections—and my dreams—since Dr. Zaki Shapira's arrest, indeed since first learning that my kidneys were once again failing, have gained focus from hindsight. The nightmare clarifies. Reality intrudes. Friendships evolve, relationships change, and life goes on inexorably. But amid all the noise, there is hardly a day that goes by without my wondering what might have happened if I had made a different decision.

I'm getting pretty adept at playing that movie in my mind.

But, really, there was no other choice.

Hopefully, this book will help enable our policy makers to develop other choices for those in need of organ transplants in the future.

I open my eyes. Outside, night has fallen. All I can see, at first, are a few wisps of clouds cut by the wings of the jet. Then, through breaks in the clouds, I see stars.

AUTHORS' NOTE

We coauthored this book to save lives. We believe the personal stories of the peasant and the power broker illuminate the problems with the growing global markets in human transplant organs and America's failed organ transplant policy. One of us contributed his story, his voice, his access to valuable sources, and his editorial comment. The other spent years following the growth of the organ markets, researching the issues, conducting the interviews, and writing the drafts and redrafts of the manuscript.

We'd like to acknowledge the valuable research assistance of Greg Boucher and Julia George. We'd also like to thank all those who sat for interviews and shared their personal stories: Ernesto Delaroca; Sandra Delaroca; Laurence Chan, MD; Igal Kam, MD; Gregg Farber; Brent Farber; Brad Farber; Lynne Sullivan; Jim Sullivan; Jimmy Lustig; Norm Brownstein; and Carolyn Abrahams. Their perspectives humanize the subject.

And, with the exceptions of some liberties taken with dialogue in the narrative sections and those needed to give the book a consistent voice, it's all true.

Harlan Abrahams
Steve Farber
Denver, January 2009

A portion of the proceeds from this book will go to the American Transplant Foundation. Please visit our Web site—www.americantransplantfoundation.org—to learn more about us.

APPENDIX A:
TRANSPLANT LAWS
AROUND THE WORLD

The following table was adapted from one prepared by the American Transplant Foundation in connection with its Forum on Transplant Tourism, held in Vail, Colorado, on March 11, 2008.

Country	Number on the national transplant waiting list	
Australia	3,000 (including tissues)	
China	1,500,000 could benefit from organ transplants each year, but only 10,000 can find compatible organs.	
India	No national registry	
Iran	No national registry	

Details

Commercial transplantation is prohibited by legislation.[1]

The Chinese government imposed new restrictions in May 2007 in an attempt to curb transplant tourism. The Health Ministry's regulations stipulate that foreigners visiting China on tourist visas cannot receive transplants, that hospitals cannot advertise abroad, and that hospitals planning to perform a transplant on a foreign patient must receive prior authorization from health authorities. Some accuse China of recovering the organs of executed prisoners in order to make organs more plentiful. Officials admit that some organs used for transplant have been from executed prisoners, but say the number of cases is low and that advance authorization is required.[2]

The Human Organ Transplant Act of 1994 bans the organ trade and states that only immediate blood relatives may become donors without government authorization.[3] After the discovery of an illegal transplant ring in Gurgaon in January 2008, the government announced that it would liberalize the current transplant laws and launch a nationwide organ awareness program, hoping to prevent the need for such illegitimate operations.[4,5] It is estimated that about 2,000 Indians sell a kidney every year.[6]

Iran adopted a unique but controversial compensated and regulated living-unrelated donor transplant program in 1988. If a patient does not have a living-related kidney donor, then he or she is matched with a volunteer donor by a government organization. After the transplant, the donor receives an award of approximately $1,200 and health insurance from the government. Due to this program, the renal transplant waiting list was eliminated in 1999. Transplant tourism has been effectively eliminated due to laws forbidding transplantation between people of different nationalities.[7]

Country	Number on the national transplant waiting list	
Japan	More than 15,000 are waiting for a kidney transplant.	
Philippines		
Saudi Arabia	More than 10,000[10]	
Spain		

	Details
	The Organ Transplant Law of 1994 permits donation from a brain-dead patient only if the donor was more than 15 years old and expressed, in writing, the intent to donate his or her organs and to agree to be submitted to brain death declarations. Family members must also approve.[8]
	Kidney sales are legal in the Philippines, where the booming transplant business draws patients from the United States, Australia, New Zealand, and Japan. The Health Ministry's program costs a foreign buyer roughly $73,700 to cover health insurance and a cash gift for the donor. The government's program is often criticized over scandals about kidney sales by slum dwellers. The organ trade is likely to increase, with the Philippine Medical Tourism Program now promoting a bill to enhance the partnership between the government and the private sector.[9]
	An October 2006 law to deter Saudi citizens from traveling to other countries to receive organ transplants states that the government will pay a "reward" (approximately $13,300) and provide lifelong medical care for unrelated organ donors. This law is implemented at the national level. After a World Health Organization meeting in November 2006, at which Saudi Arabia and 13 other countries from the eastern Mediterranean region pledged to oppose the commercialization of organ donation, Saudi authorities were considering how to make this agreement altruistic, with donors receiving rewards, not cash. Prior to the new law, only patients who were declared brain dead and immediate family members were allowed to donate organs.[11]
	Spain, a country with presumed consent (Law No. 30 of 1979), has the highest donation rates in the world. Though not explicitly required by law, in practice, organs are used only with permission of the donors' families. The Transplantation Act of 1980 protects the altruistic character of organ donation and forbids organ marketing.[12]

Country	Number on the national transplant waiting list
United Kingdom	More than 9,000[13]
United States of America	More than 98,000

	Details
	Laws in the United Kingdom forbid the commercialization of organs for transplant. In January 2008, Prime Minister Gordon Brown proposed a national debate about changing British laws to adopt a presumed consent system to increase organ donations.[14]
	The National Organ Transplant Act of 1984 makes it a crime to engage in organ sale and commerce for the purpose of transplantation. However, it is legal to sell organs and tissues for the purpose of research.[15]

APPENDIX B:
NATIONAL ORGAN
TRANSPLANT ACT

(As amended by the Charlie W. Norwood Living Organ Donation Act—January 2008)

Sec. 273.—Organ procurement organizations

(a) Grant authority of Secretary

(1) The Secretary may make grants for the planning of qualified organ procurement organizations described in subsection (b) of this section.

(2) The Secretary may make grants for the establishment, initial operation, consolidation, and expansion of qualified organ procurement organizations described in subsection (b) of this section.

(3) The Secretary may make grants to, and enter into contracts with, qualified organ procurement organizations described in subsection (b) of this section and other nonprofit private entities for the purpose of carrying out special projects designed to increase the number of organ donors.

(b) Qualified organizations

(1) A qualified organ procurement organization for which grants may be made under subsection (a) of this section is an organization which, as determined by the Secretary, will carry out the functions described in paragraph (2) and –

(A) is a nonprofit entity,

(B) has accounting and other fiscal procedures (as specified by the Secretary) necessary to assure the fiscal stability of the organization,

(C) has an agreement with the Secretary to be reimbursed under title XVIII of the Social Security Act (42 U.S.C. 1395 et seq.) for the procurement of kidneys,

(D) notwithstanding any other provision of law, has met the other requirements of this section and has been certified or recertified by the Secretary within the previous 4-year period as meeting the performance standards to be a qualified organ procurement organization through a process that either –

(i) granted certification or recertification within such 4-year period with such certification or recertification in effect as of January 1, 2000, and remaining in effect through the earlier of –

(I) January 1, 2002; or

(II) the completion of recertification under the requirements of clause (ii); or

(ii) is defined through regulations that are promulgated by the Secretary by not later than January 1, 2002, that –

(I) require recertifications of qualified organ procurement organizations not more frequently than once every 4 years;

(II) rely on outcome and process performance

measures that are based on empirical evidence, obtained through reasonable efforts, of organ donor potential and other related factors in each service area of qualified organ procurement organizations;

(III) use multiple outcome measures as part of the certification process; and

(IV) provide for a qualified organ procurement organization to appeal a decertification to the Secretary on substantive and procedural grounds;

(E) has procedures to obtain payment for non-renal organs provided to transplant centers,

(F) has a defined service area that is of sufficient size to assure maximum effectiveness in the procurement and equitable distribution of organs, and that either includes an entire metropolitan statistical area (as specified by the Director of the Office of Management and Budget) or does not include any part of the area,

(G) has a director and such other staff, including the organ donation coordinators and organ procurement specialists necessary to effectively obtain organs from donors in its service area, and

(H) has a board of directors or an advisory board which –

(i) is composed of -

(I) members who represent hospital administrators, intensive care or emergency room personnel, tissue banks, and voluntary health associations in its service area,

(II) members who represent the public residing in such area,

(III) a physician with knowledge, experience, or skill in the field of histocompatability or an individual with a doctorate degree in a biological science with knowledge, experience, or skill in the field of histocompatibility, "histocompatibility,"

(IV) physician with knowledge or skill in the field of neurology, and

(V) from each transplant center in its service area which has arrangements described in paragraph (2)(G) with the organization, a member who is a surgeon who has practicing privileges in such center and who performs organ transplant surgery,

(ii) has the authority to recommend policies for the procurement of organs and the other functions described in paragraph (2), and

(iii) has no authority over any other activity of the organization.

(2)

(A) Not later than 90 days after November 16, 1990, the Secretary shall publish in the Federal Register a notice of proposed rulemaking to establish criteria for determining whether an entity meets the requirement established in paragraph (1)(E).

(B) Not later than 1 year after November 16, 1990, the Secretary shall publish in the Federal Register a final rule to establish the criteria described in subparagraph (A).

(3) An organ procurement organization shall –

(A) have effective agreements, to identify potential organ donors, with a substantial majority of the hospitals and other health care entities in its service area which have facilities for organ donations,

(B) conduct and participate in systematic efforts, including professional education, to acquire all useable organs from potential donors,

(C) arrange for the acquisition and preservation of donated organs and provide quality standards for the acquisition of organs which are consistent with the standards adopted by the Organ Procurement and Transplantation Network under section 274(b)(2)(E) of this title, including arranging for testing with respect to preventing the acquisition of organs that are infected with the etiologic agent for acquired immune deficiency syndrome,

(D) arrange for the appropriate tissue typing of donated organs,

(E) have a system to allocate donated organs equitably among transplant patients according to established medical criteria,

(F) provide or arrange for the transportation of donated organs to transplant centers,

(G) have arrangements to coordinate its activities with transplant centers in its service area,

(H) participate in the Organ Procurement Transplantation Network established under section 274 of this title,

(I) have arrangements to cooperate with tissue banks for the retrieval, processing, preservation, storage, and distribution of tissues as may be appropriate to assure that all useable tissues are obtained from potential donors,

(J) evaluate annually the effectiveness of the organization in acquiring potentially available organs, and

(K) assist hospitals in establishing and implementing protocols for making routine inquiries about organ donations by potential donors

Sec. 274.—Organ procurement and transplantation network

(a) Contract authority of Secretary; limitation; available appropriations

The Secretary shall by contract provide for the establishment and operation of an Organ Procurement and Transplantation Network which meets the requirements of subsection (b) of this section. The amount provided under such contract in any fiscal year may not exceed $2,000,000. Funds for such contracts shall be made available from funds available to the Public Health Service from appropriations for fiscal years beginning after fiscal year 1984.

(b) Functions

(1) The Organ Procurement and Transplantation Network shall carry out the functions described in paragraph (2) and shall –

(A) be a private nonprofit entity that has an expertise in organ procurement and transplantation, and

(B) have a board of directors –

> (i) that includes representatives of organ procurement organizations (including organizations that have received grants under section 273 of this title), transplant centers, voluntary health associations, and the general public; and

> (ii) that shall establish an executive committee and other committees, whose chairpersons shall be selected to ensure continuity of leadership for the board.

(2) The Organ Procurement and Transplantation Network shall –

(A) establish in one location or through regional centers –

> (i) a national list of individuals who need organs, and

> (ii) a national system, through the use of computers and in accordance with established medical criteria, to match organs and individuals included in the list, especially individuals whose immune system makes it difficult for them to receive organs,

(B) establish membership criteria and medical criteria for allocating organs and provide to members of the public an opportunity to comment with respect to such criteria,

(C) maintain a twenty-four-hour telephone service to facilitate matching organs with individuals included in the list,

(D) assist organ procurement organizations in the nationwide distribution of organs equitably among transplant patients,

(E) adopt and use standards of quality for the acquisition and transportation of donated organs, including standards for preventing the acquisition of organs that are infected with the etiologic agent for acquired immune deficiency syndrome,

(F) prepare and distribute, on a regionalized basis (and, to the extent practicable, among regions or on a national basis), samples of blood sera from individuals who are included on the list and whose immune system makes it difficult for them to receive organs, in order to facilitate matching the compatibility of such individuals with organ donors,

(G) coordinate, as appropriate, the transportation of organs from organ procurement organizations to transplant centers,

(H) provide information to physicians and other health professionals regarding organ donation,

(I) collect, analyze, and publish data concerning organ donation and transplants,

(J) carry out studies and demonstration projects for the purpose of improving procedures for organ procurement and allocation,

(K) work actively to increase the supply of donated organs,

(L) submit to the Secretary an annual report containing information on the comparative costs and patient outcomes at each transplant center affiliated with the organ procurement and transplantation network,

(M) recognize the differences in health and in organ transplantation issues between children and adults throughout the system and adopt criteria, policies, and procedures that address the unique health care needs of children,

(N) carry out studies and demonstration projects for the purpose of improving procedures for organ donation procurement and allocation, including but not limited to projects to examine and attempt to increase transplantation among populations with special needs, including children and individuals who are members of racial or ethnic minority groups, and among populations with limited access to transportation, and

(O) provide that for purposes of this paragraph, the term "children" refers to individuals who are under the age of 18.

(c) Consideration of critical comments

The Secretary shall establish procedures for –

(1) receiving from interested persons critical comments relating to the manner in which the Organ Procurement and Transplantation Network is carrying out the duties of the Network under subsection (b) of this section; and

(2) the consideration by the Secretary of such critical comments

Sec. 274a.—Scientific registry

The Secretary shall, by grant or contract, develop and maintain a scientific registry of the recipients of organ transplants. The registry shall include such information respecting patients and transplant procedures as the Secretary deems necessary to an ongoing evaluation of the scientific and clinical status of organ transplantation. The Secretary shall prepare for inclusion in the report under section 274d of this title an analysis of information derived from the registry.

Sec. 274b.—General provisions respecting grants and contracts

(a) Application requirement

No grant may be made under this part or contract entered into under section 274 or 274a of this title unless an application therefore has been submitted to, and approved by, the Secretary. Such an application shall be in such form and shall be submitted in such manner as the Secretary shall by regulation prescribe.

(b) Special considerations and priority; planning and establishment grants

(1)   A grant for planning under section 273(a)(1) of this title may be made for one year with respect to any organ procurement organization and may not exceed $100,000.

(2)   Grants under section 273(a)(2) of this title may be made for two years. No such grant may exceed $500,000 for any year and no organ procurement organization may receive more than $800,000 for initial operation or expansion.

(3)   Grants or contracts under section 273(a)(3) of this title may be made for not more than 3 years.

(c) Determination of grant amount; terms of payment; recordkeeping; access for purposes of audits and examination of records

(1) The Secretary shall determine the amount of a grant or contract made under section 273 or 274a of this title. Payments under such grants and contracts may be made in advance on the basis of estimates or by the way of reimbursement, with necessary adjustments on account of underpayments or overpayments, and in such installments and on such terms and conditions as the Secretary finds necessary to carry out the purposes of such grants and contracts.

(2)

    (A) Each recipient of a grant or contract under section 273 or 274a of this title shall keep such records as the Secretary shall prescribe, including records which fully disclose the amount and disposition by such recipient of the proceeds of such grant or contract, the total cost of the undertaking in connection with which such grant or contract was made, and the amount of that portion of the cost of the undertaking supplied by other sources, and such other records as will facilitate an effective audit.

    (B) The Secretary and the Comptroller General of the United States, or any of their duly authorized representatives, shall have access for the purpose of audit and examination to any books, documents, papers, and records of the recipient of a grant or contract under section 273 or 274a of this title that are pertinent to such grant or contract.

(d) "Transplant center" and "organ" defined

For purposes of this part:

(1) The term "transplant center" means a health care facility in which transplants of organs are performed.

(2) The term "organ" means the human kidney, liver, heart,

lung, pancreas, and any other human organ (other than corneas and eyes) specified by the Secretary by regulation and for purposes of section 274a of this title, such term includes bone marrow

Sec. 274c.—Administration

The Secretary shall designate and maintain an identifiable administrative unit in the Public Health Service to –

(1) administer this part and coordinate with the organ procurement activities under title XVIII of the Social Security Act (42 U.S.C. 1395 et seq.),

(2) conduct a program of public information to inform the public of the need for organ donations,

(3) provide technical assistance to organ procurement organizations, the Organ Procurement and Transplantation Network established under section 274 of this title, and other entities in the health care system involved in organ donations, procurement, and transplants, and

(4) provide information –

   (i) to patients, their families, and their physicians about transplantation; and

   (ii) to patients and their families about the resources available nationally and in each State, and the comparative costs and patient outcomes at each transplant center affiliated with the organ procurement and transplantation network, in order to assist the patients and families with the costs associated with transplantation

Sec. 274d.—Report

Not later than February 10 of 1991 and of each second year thereafter, the Secretary shall publish, and submit to the Committee on Energy and Commerce of the House of Representatives and the Committee on Labor and Human Resources of the Senate a report on the scientific and clinical status of organ transplantation. The Secretary shall consult with the Director of the National Institutes of Health and the Commissioner of the Food and Drug Administration in the preparation of the report.

Sec. 274e.—Prohibition of organ purchases

(a) Prohibition

It shall be unlawful for any person to knowingly acquire, receive, or otherwise transfer any human organ for valuable consideration for use in human transplantation if the transfer affects interstate commerce. The preceding sentence does not apply with respect to human organ paired donation.

(b) Penalties

Any person who violates subsection (a) of this section shall be fined not more than $50,000 or imprisoned not more than five years, or both.

(c) Definitions

For purposes of subsection (a) of this section:

(1) The term "human organ" means the human (including fetal) kidney, liver, heart, lung, pancreas, bone marrow, cornea, eye, bone, and skin or any subpart thereof and any other human organ (or any subpart thereof, including that derived from a fetus) specified by the Secretary of Health and Human Services by regulation.

(2) The term "valuable consideration" does not include the reasonable payments associated with the removal, transportation, implantation, processing, preservation, quality control, and storage of a human organ or the expenses of travel, housing, and lost wages incurred by the donor of a human organ in connection with the donation of the organ.

(3) The term "interstate commerce" has the meaning prescribed for it by section 321(b) of title 21

(4) The term "human organ paired donation" means the donation and receipt of human organs under the following circumstances:

(A) An individual (referred to in this paragraph as the "first donor") desires to make a living donation of a human organ specifically to a particular patient (referred to in this paragraph as the "first patient"), but such donor is biologically incompatible as a donor for such patient.

(B) A second individual (referred to in this paragraph as the "second donor") desires to make a living donation of a human organ specifically to a second particular patient (referred to in this paragraph as the "second patient"), but such donor is biologically incompatible as a donor for such patient.

(C) Subject to subparagraph (D), the first donor is biologically compatible as a donor of a human organ for the second patient, and the second donor is biologically compatible as a donor of a human organ for the first patient.

(D) If there is any additional donor-patient pair as described in subparagraph (A) or (B), each donor in the group of donor-patient pairs is biologically compatible as a donor of a human organ for a patient in such group.

(E) All donors and patients in the group of donor-patient pairs (whether 2 pairs or more than 2 pairs) enter into a single agreement to donate and receive such human organs, respectively, according to such biological compatibility in the group.

(F) Other than as described in subparagraph (E), no valuable consideration is knowingly acquired, received, or otherwise transferred with respect to the human organs referred to in such subparagraph.

Sec. 274f.—Study by General Accounting Office

(a) In general

The Comptroller General of the United States shall conduct a study for the purpose of determining –

(1) the extent to which the procurement and allocation of organs have been equitable, efficient, and effective;

(2) the problems encountered in the procurement and allocation; and

(3) the effect of State required-request laws.

(b) Report

Not later than January 7, 1992, the Comptroller General of the United States shall complete the study required in subsection (a) of this section and submit to the Committee on Energy and Commerce of the House of Representatives, and to the Committee on Labor and Human Resources of the Senate, a report describing the findings made as a result of the study.

Sec. 274g.—Authorization of appropriations

For the purpose of carrying out this part, there are authorized to be appropriated $8,000,000 for fiscal year 1991, and such sums as may be necessary for each of the fiscal years 1992 and 1993.

ENDNOTES

Prologue

1 Many Internet Web sites covered the arrest. The accounts that were consulted in the writing of the Prologue included: "Shoot-out at Transplant Hospital Lands Israeli Surgeon in Jail," *BioEdge* 250, May 23, 2007, http://www.australasianbioethics.org/Newsletters/250-2007-05-23.html; "Israeli Doctor Said Detained in Turkey for Illegal Organ Transplants," Haaretz.com, May 1, 2007, http://www.haaretz.com/hasen/spages/854612.html; "Israeli Suspected of Organ Trafficking," *Jerusalem Post*, May 2, 2007, http://www.jpost.com/servlet/Satellite?pagename=JPost/JPArticle/ShowFull&cid=1178020745802; Lilach Shoval, "Turkey Arrests Israeli Suspected of Organ Trafficking," YNetNews.com, May 1, 2007, http://www.ynetnews.com/articles/0,7340,L-3394513,00.html; Merav Sarig, "Israeli Transplant Surgeon Is Arrested for Suspected Organ Trafficking," *British Medical Journal* 334:973, May 12, 2007, http://www.bmj.com/cgi/content/extract/334/7601/973; "Israeli Suspected of Organ Trading," Press TV, May 2, 2007, http://www.presstv.ir/detail.aspx?id=8347&sectionid=3510212; and "Israeli Doctor Arrested in Turkey on Suspicion of Trafficking Human Organs," Ma'an News Agency, May 2, 2007, http://www.maannews.net/en/index.php?opr=ShowDetails&ID=21711.

Chapter One

1 The sources consulted for background and information included: "José Efraín Ríos Montt," The Free Dictionary, http://www.encyclopedia.thefreedictionary.com/Rios%20Montt; and "Efrain Rios Montt," Third World Traveler, http://www.thirdworldtraveler.com/Zeroes/Efrain_Rios_Montt.html.

2 One estimate of approximately 600 was reported at "José Efraín Ríos Montt," The Free Dictionary.

3 This statistic is reported at "Efrain Rios Montt," Third World Traveler. Unfortunately, President Ronald Reagan was a big

supporter of the Guatemalan tyrant. His praise is quoted at "Efrain Rios Montt," Third World Traveler.

4 The rules governing organ allocation favor rural states because, when a cadaveric organ becomes available, proximity is one of the principal factors that determines who gets the organ. So, if an organ becomes available in a sparsely populated rural area, a nearby rural recipient who is lower on the waiting list will receive the organ instead of potential recipients who are higher on the waiting list but are located in urban areas that are too far away under the rules. For the many factors used in allocating organs, see Department of Health and Human Services, "Organ Procurement and Transplantation Network Final Rule," *Code of Federal Regulations* 42, Part 121, October 20, 1999, http://www.optn.org/downloadables/final_rule.pdf. See also Organ Procurement and Transplantation Network, "Members: Regions," http://www.optn.org/members/regions/asp, for discussion of why organs are offered first to those located in the region where the death of the donor occurs. Major revisions to the rules concerning organ allocation have been proposed, and some have been adopted, as is discussed more fully in Chapter Eleven.

5 The federal prohibition is set forth in the National Organ Transplant Act, which has been codified at *United States Code* 42, Section 274e(a); the prohibitions in state laws are usually worded similarly and found in the states' variations on the Uniform Anatomical Gift Act (UAGA), which all 50 have adopted in some form or another. Recently, a Revised Uniform Anatomical Gift Act has been promulgated and is in the process of being adopted by the states. Provisions in the revised UAGA and recent amendments to the federal statute are discussed more fully in Chapter Eleven.

6 Justice Stanley Mosk, dissenting in the California Supreme Court case of *Moore v. Regents of the University of California*, 793 P.2d 479, 517–518, 1991, explained this odd reality:

As to organs, the majority rely on the Uniform Anatomical Gift Act [UAGA] . . . for the proposition that a competent adult may make a postmortem gift of any part of his body but may not receive "valuable consideration" for the transfer. But the prohibition of the UAGA against the sale of a body part is much more limited than the majority recognize: by its terms . . . the prohibition applies only to sales for "transplantation" or "therapy." Yet a different section of the UAGA authorizes the transfer and receipt of body parts for such additional purposes as "medical or dental education, research, or advancement of medical or dental science. . . . " No section of the UAGA prohibits anyone from selling body parts for any of those additional purposes; by clear implication, . . . such sales are legal. Indeed, the fact that the UAGA prohibits *no* sales of organs other than sales for "transplantation" or "therapy" raises a further implication that it is also legal for anyone to sell human tissue to a biotechnology company for research and development purposes.

7 The UAGA applies, for example, only to postmortem donations. *Uniform Laws Annotated* 8A, 19, 1993.

8 Public Law No. 98-507, 98 Stat. 2339, 1984, codified at *United States Code* 42, sections 273–274, also known as the National Organ Transplant Act of 1984 (NOTA as amended through May 2008). NOTA is the key to American transplant policy. Recent amendments to NOTA are discussed in Chapter Eleven. The statute is reprinted in its entirety in Appendix B.

9 The data come from the Web sites of the United Network for Organ Sharing (UNOS; www.unos.org) and the Organ Procurement and Transplantation Network (www.optn.org), both of which contain a wealth of statistics, information, and resources. Some are updated continuously. For example, at 11:22 a.m. EDT on May 7, 2008, there were 99,195 people on the official waiting list, of whom 75,836 were waiting for kidneys. On average, 18 patients die each day while waiting for an organ, totaling roughly 6,570 people each year. See United Network for Organ Sharing, "Resources: Publications: Fact Sheets," July 20, 2005, http://www.unos.org/resources/factsheets.asp?fs=3. UNOS announced that the list for kidneys first exceeded 60,000 on October 14, 2004. See United Network for Organ Sharing, "Kidney Transplant Need Exceeds 60,000," October 14, 2007, www.unos.org/news/newsDetail.asp?id=358.

10   See Debra Satz, "Noxious Markets: Why Should Some
Things Not Be for Sale?" in Stephen Cullenberg and
Prasanta K. Pattanaik, editors, *Globalization, Culture, and
the Limits of the Market* (Oxford, England: Oxford University
Press, 2003), p. 32.

11   Live kidney sales are legal in Iran, even though cadaveric
donations are not allowed due to Iran's strict fundamentalist
interpretation of Islamic law. The Charity Association for the
Support of Kidney Patients and the Charity Foundation for
Special Diseases are both nongovernmental organizations that
facilitate the kidney trade in Iran. Both are endorsed and fully
regulated by the country's Islamic government. See Sheera
Frenkel, "Organ-Trafficking Laws in Key Countries," *Christian
Science Monitor* June 9, 2004, http://www.csmonitor.
com/2004/0609/p12s02-wogi.html.

12   The concept or process of "commodification" is essential to the
work of the Free Market Camp. David Kaserman, one of the
more prominent champions of the Free Market Camp, has
written many articles and coauthored a book to promote the idea.
See David L. Kaserman and A. H. Barnett, *The U.S. Organ
Procurement System: A Prescription for Reform* (Washington, DC:
American Enterprise Institute Press, 2002).

13   The Human Rights Camp is led by University of California–
Berkeley professor Nancy Scheper-Hughes, cofounder of the
nonprofit group Organs Watch. She testified in detail before
Congress on June 27, 2001, and has written extensively on the
subject of trafficking in organs. Her work is critical to any
evaluation of the growing global markets for organs. It is cited
throughout this book and much of it is reproduced on the Organs
Watch Web site, http://sunsite3.berkeley.edu/biotech/
organswatch.

14   For an excellent summary of the basic attributes of political
sovereignty in the new millennium, see Maryann Cusimano
Love, *Beyond Sovereignty: Issues for a Global Agenda* (Belmont,
California: Thomson/Wadsworth, 2003), p. 3. This is one of the
earliest and best of the academic book-length treatments focusing
on the intersections and conflicts between the economics of
globalization and the politics of sovereignty.

Chapter Two

1 The sources consulted for this brief summary of the history of transplant medicine included: Peter Medawar, *Memoir of a Thinking Radish: An Autobiography* (Oxford, England: Oxford University Press, 1988); Roy Calne, *A Gift of Life: Observations on Organ Transplantation* (New York: Basic Books, 1970); Roy Calne, *The Ultimate Gift: The Story of Britain's Premier Transplant Surgeon* (London: Headline, 1998); "Roy Calne Biography (1930–)," How Products Are Made, http://www.madehow.com/inventorbios/66/Roy-Calne.html; New York Organ Donor Network, "History of Organ Transplantation," http://www.donatelifeny.org/transplant/organ_history.html; Lawrence K. Altman, "The Ultimate Gift: 50 Years of Organ Transplants," *New York Times* December 21, 2004, http://www.nytimes.com/2004/12/21/health/21orga.html; "Organ Transplant," Wikipedia, http://en.wikipedia.org/wiki/Organ_transplantation; and United Network for Organ Sharing, "Who We Are: History," http://www.unos.org/whoweare/history.asp.

2 Peter Boyles, "Q&A: Steve Farber & Norm Brownstein," *5280* April 2003, p. 136.

Chapter Three

1 Austen Garwood-Gowers, *Living Donor Organ Transplantation: Key Legal and Ethical Issues* (Aldershot, England: Ashgate, 1999), p. 6.

2 See Garwood-Gowers, *Living Donor Organ Transplantation.*

3 Although the Supreme Court has never squarely addressed the issue, it has addressed closely analogous issues many times. For one of the more recent and more definitive cases, see generally *Cruzan v. Director, Missouri Department of Health*, US 497:261, 1990 (Chief Justice William Rehnquist, writing the majority opinion, explained: "For purposes of this case, we assume that the United States Constitution would grant a competent person a constitutionally protected right to refuse lifesaving hydration and nutrition"); see also *Stamford Hospital v. Vega*, 674 A.2d 821 (Conn. 1996).

4 See generally *Employment Division, Department of Human Resources of Oregon v. Smith*, U.S. 494:872, 1990; see also *People v. Woody*, 61 Cal.2d 716, 1964.

5 *Griswold v. Connecticut*, U.S. 381:479, 1965. The quoted language is part of a longer passage at p. 484 in the majority opinion written by Justice William O. Douglas, which is often quoted in its entirety:

> The . . . cases suggest that specific guarantees in the Bill of Rights have penumbras, formed by emanations from those guarantees that help give them life and substance. See *Poe v. Ullman*, 367 U.S. 497, 516-22 (1961)(dissenting opinion). Various guarantees create zones of privacy. The right of association contained in the penumbra of the First Amendment is one, as we have seen. The Third Amendment in its prohibition against the quartering of soldiers "in any house" in time of peace without the consent of the owner is another facet of that privacy. The Fourth Amendment explicitly affirms the "right of the people to be secure in their persons, houses, papers, and effects, against unreasonable searches and seizures." The Fifth Amendment in its Self-Incrimination Clause enables the citizen to create a zone of privacy which government may not force him to surrender to his detriment. The Ninth Amendment provides: "The enumeration in the Constitution, of certain rights shall not be construed to deny or disparage others retained by the people."

> The Fourth and Fifth Amendments were described in Boyd v. United States, U.S. 116:616, 1886, as protection against all governmental invasions "of the sanctity of a man's home and the privacies of life." We recently referred in Mapp v. Ohio, U.S. 367:643, 1961, to the Fourth Amendment as creating a "right to privacy, no less important than any other right carefully and particularly reserved to the people."

> The present case, then, concerns a relationship lying within the zone of privacy created by several fundamental constitutional guarantees.

6 *Roe v. Wade*, U.S. 410:113, 153, 1973. Like its predecessor in *Griswold*, the Supreme Court in *Roe* faced circumstances inextricably intertwined with human reproduction and the integrity of a woman's body. Interestingly, it was a fairly

conservative justice—Harry Blackmun, appointed by a Republican—who wrote the majority opinion. The language quoted in the text comes from the following longer passage, p. 153 in the majority opinion:

> The Constitution does not explicitly mention any right of privacy. In a [long] line of cases, however . . . the Court has recognized that a right of personal privacy, or a guarantee of certain areas or zones of privacy, does exist under the Constitution. In varying contexts, the Court or individual Justices have, indeed, found at least the roots of that right in the First Amendment; or in the concept of liberty guaranteed by the first section of the Fourteenth Amendment. These decisions make it clear that only personal rights that can be deemed "fundamental" or "implicit in the concept of ordered liberty," *Palko v. Connecticut*, are included in this guarantee of personal privacy. They also make it clear that the right has some extension to activities relating to marriage, *Loving v. Virginia*; procreation, *Skinner v. Oklahoma*; contraception, *Eisenstadt v. Baird*; family relationships, *Prince v. Massachusetts*; and child rearing and education, *Pierce v. Society of Sisters, Meyer v. Nebraska*.
>
> This right of privacy, whether it be found in the Fourteenth Amendment's concept of personal liberty and restrictions upon state action, as we feel it is, or, as the District court determined, the Ninth Amendment's reservation of rights to the people, is broad enough to encompass a woman's decision whether or not to terminate her pregnancy.

7 See *Lawrence v. Texas*, U.S. 539:538, 2003, overruling *Bowers v. Hardwick*, U.S. 478:178, 1986.

8 *Lawrence v. Texas*, U.S. 539:562. Ironically, it was once again a conservative justice—this time Anthony Kennedy—who wrote for the majority, extending the right of privacy beyond its prior boundaries.

9 Cusimano Love, *Beyond Sovereignty*, p. 3.

10 H. Abrahams and J. Snowden, "Separation of Powers and Administrative Crimes: A Study of Irreconcilables," *Southern*

Illinois University Law Journal 1:22, 1976 (also, "social forces were forming the setting for a redefining of sovereignty").

11 Thomas L. Friedman, *Longitudes and Attitudes: Exploring the World After September 11* (New York: Farrar, Strauss and Giroux, 2002), p. 3; see also Thomas L. Friedman, *The Lexus and the Olive Tree: Understanding Globalization* (New York: Anchor Books, 2000), p. 9. In *Longitudes and Attitudes*, p. 9, Friedman elaborates: "The driving force behind globalization is free market capitalism—the more you let market forces rule and the more you open your economy to free trade and competition, the more efficient and flourishing your economy will be. Globalization means the spread of free-market capitalism to virtually every country in the world." In a similar way, in *Globalization and Its Discontents* (New York: W. W. Norton, 2003), Columbia University professor Joseph E. Stiglitz, winner of the Nobel Prize in Economics, defines globalization as "the closer integration of the countries and peoples of the world which has been brought about by the enormous reduction of costs of transportation and communication, and the breaking down of artificial barriers to the free flow of goods, services, capital, knowledge, and (to a lesser extent) people across borders." Whichever definition is used, it's clear that "globalization," as the term is commonly used today, is first and foremost an economic phenomenon that involves the spread of free market capitalism throughout the world in one form or another. And the inevitable clash between that economic phenomenon and the political forces of sovereignty is plainly foreshadowed in the final two words in Stiglitz's definition: "across borders."

Chapter Four

1 National Organ Transplant Act, Section 274e, Appendix B.

2 Pennsylvania offers several hundred dollars toward funeral expenses if the family of a decedent allows the deceased's body to be used for organ donation. *Pennsylvania Consolidated Statutes* 20, Section 8622, 1999. Furthermore, according to "Organ and Tissue Donation and Transplantation: A Legal Perspective" from the National Attorneys' Committee for Transplant Awareness (posted at http://www.lawsmart.com/documents/

orgdonr1.shtml): "Eighteen states have enacted medical examiner's laws that presume consent of a decedent in certain limited circumstances. However, these laws are generally very limited in scope, and in some states are encountering opposition from those who believe they violate one's Constitutional right to privacy." Other notable experiments by several states, as well as the debates over presumed consent, are discussed in Chapter Eleven.

3 The Organs Watch Web site can be found at http://sunsite. berkeley.edu/biotech/organswatch. The Web site includes or links to volumes of valuable data and opinions, but it has not been updated for some time.

4 Nancy Scheper-Hughes, "The Ends of the Body: The Global Commerce in Organs for Transplant Surgery," http://sunsite. berkeley.edu/biotech/organswatch/pages/endsofbody.html.

5 Nancy Scheper-Hughes, "The Global Traffic in Human Organs: A Report Presented to the House Subcommittee on International Operations and Human Rights, United States Congress, June 27, 2001," http://www.publicanthropology.org/ TimesPast/Scheper-Hughes.htm.

6 See Nancy Scheper-Hughes, "The Organ of Last Resort," *UNESCO Courier* July/August 2001, http://www.unesco.org/ courier/2001_07/uk/doss34.htm; and Scheper-Hughes, "The Global Traffic in Human Organs."

7 Karl Marx, *Das Kapital*, Chapter Three.

8 Richard D. Lamm, *The Brave New World of Health Care* (Golden, Colorado: Fulcrum, 2003), p. 37.

9 The final rule can be found in its entirety at http://www.optn. org/downloadables/final_rule.pdf. As mentioned previously, these rules and regulations are in a constant state of revision.

10 For four surveys of the different religious views on organ donation, see East Tennessee Lions Eye Bank, "Religious Views Concerning Organ and Tissue Donation," http://www. discoveret.org/eyebank/religious.html; Gift of Life Foundation, "Religious Views on Organ Donation and Transplantation," http://www.giftoflifefoundation.com; Center for Donation and

Transplant, "Religious Views on Donation," http://cdtny.org/donation-religion; and Transplant for Life, "Your Religion," www.transplantforlife.org/miracles/religion.html.

11 See East Tennessee Lions Eye Bank, "Religious Views Concerning Organ and Tissue Donation."

12 East Tennessee Lions Eye Bank, "Religious Views Concerning Organ and Tissue Donation." Jews nevertheless have some of the lowest donation rates among religious and ethnic groups. Some say this is because many Jews question the medical concept of brain death. Others see a different reason:

> [T]here is also . . . the very real halachic concept of *kavod hamet*, preserving the dignity of the body that housed the departed soul.
> Cadavers are treated with honor, so that modesty is retained even during the ritual washing. The body is never left alone, and it is buried as soon as possible. . . .
> But everyone involved in the halachic debate surrounding organ donation agrees that all those laws must be overridden if it is a matter of *pikuach nefesh*, saving a life—considered one of the greatest mitzvot in Judaism, surpassing most commands.

See also Julie Gruenbaum Fax, "Reluctance to Donate Organs Persists, Despite New Views," *Jewish News Weekly of Northern California* February 27, 2004, http://www.jewishsf.com (search for "donate organs").

13 See A. A. Sachedina, "Islamic Views on Organ Transplantation," *Transplantation Proceedings* 20(1 Suppl 1):1084–1088, 1988, quoted in J. McCarthy, "Organ Donation: A Catholic and Interfaith Perspective on Its Ethical Warrants and Contemporary Public Policy Concerns," in William R. DeLong, editor, *Organ Transplantation in Religious, Ethical, and Social Context: No Room for Death* (New York: Haworth Pastoral Press, 1993), p. 114. Fundamentalist Muslims, like many Orthodox Jews, remain relatively resistant to cadaveric donations, however.

14 See East Tennessee Lions Eye Bank, "Religious Views Concerning Organ and Tissue Donation"; Gift of Life Foundation, "Religious Views on Organ Donation and Transplantation";

Center for Donation and Transplant, "Religious Views on Donation"; and Transplant for Life, "Your Religion."

15 See East Tennessee Lions Eye Bank, "Religious Views Concerning Organ and Tissue Donation."

16 See Gift of Life Foundation, "Religious Views on Organ Donation and Transplantation."

17 Arthur L. Caplan and Daniel H. Coelho, editors, *The Ethics of Organ Transplants: The Current Debate* (Amherst, NY: Prometheus Books, 1998).

18 See generally Austen Garwood-Gowers, *Living Donor Organ Transplantation: Key Legal and Ethical Issues* (Aldershot, England: Ashgate, 1999); Stuart J. Youngner, Renée C. Fox, and Laurence J. O'Connell, editors, *Organ Transplantation: Meanings and Realities* (Madison, Wisconsin: University of Wisconsin Press, 1996); Ronald Munson, *Raising the Dead: Organ Transplants, Ethics, and Society* (Oxford, England: Oxford University Press, 2002); David Price, *Legal and Ethical Aspects of Organ Transplantation* (Cambridge, England: Cambridge University Press, 2000); David L. Kaserman and A. H. Barnett, *The U.S. Organ Procurement System: A Prescription for Reform* (Washington, DC: American Enterprise Institute Press, 2002); Nora Machado, *Using the Bodies of the Dead: Legal, Ethical, and Organisational Dimensions of Organ Transplantation* (Aldershot, England: Ashgate, 1998); David Lamb, *Organ Transplants and Ethics* (New York: Routledge, 1990); and Robert M. Veatch, *Transplantation Ethics* (Washington, DC: Georgetown University Press, 2000).

19 *See* H. T. Engelhardt Jr., "Giving, Selling, and Having Taken: Conflicting Views of Organ Transfer," *Indiana Health Law Review* 1:31–49, 2004.

Chapter Five

1 Nancy Scheper-Hughes, "The Global Traffic in Human Organs: A Report Presented to the House Subcommittee on International Operations and Human Rights, United States Congress, June 27, 2001," http://www.publicanthropology.org/TimesPast/Scheper-Hughes.htm.

2   Scheper-Hughes, "The Global Traffic in Human Organs."

3   Debra Satz, "Noxious Markets: Why Should Some Things Not
    Be for Sale?" in Stephen Cullenberg and Prasanta K. Pattanaik,
    editors, *Globalization, Culture, and the Limits of the Market*
    (Oxford, England: Oxford University Press, 2003), p. 36.

4   The blog by authors and economists Stephen J. Dubner and
    Steven D. Levitt is easily accessed at http://freakonomics.blogs.
    nytimes.com. A cursory search shows that topics related to organ
    transplants and market-based solutions to organ shortages have
    appeared dozens of times in the past several years. While the
    authors appear to hold back from openly endorsing market
    solutions and do tend to present both sides of the arguments,
    their orientation leans toward solutions grounded in economics
    and market incentives. Some of their blogs on the subject include:
    Stephen J. Dubner, "Human Organs for Sale, Legally, in . . .
    Which Country?" April 29, 2008; Stephen J. Dubner, "Is the
    Ground Shifting for Organ Donation?" October 23, 2006; and
    Stephen J. Dubner, "Is America Ready for an Organ-Donor
    Market?" May 15, 2006; see also Stephen J. Dubner and Steven
    D. Levitt, "Flesh Trade: Weighing the Repugnance Factor," *New
    York Times Magazine* July 9, 2006, http:/www.nytimes.
    com/2006/07/09/magazine/09wwln_freak.html.

5   H. Hansmann, "The Economics and Ethics of Markets for
    Human Organs," quoted in James F. Blumstein and Frank A.
    Sloan, editors, *Organ Transplantation Policy: Issues and Prospects*
    (Durham, North Carolina: Duke University Press, 1989).

6   See generally Richard A. Posner, *Economic Analysis of Law* (New
    York: Aspen, 1998); and Milton Friedman, *Price Theory* (Chi-
    cago: Aldine, 1976). During the 1970s and 1980s, the law and
    economics movement, often seen as aligned with the political
    Right, was battled by the critical legal studies movement, often
    seen as aligned with the Left. See H. Abrahams, "The Emer-
    gence of Critical Social Theory in American Jurisprudence,"
    University of Puget Sound Law Review 4:39, 1980. The critical
    legal studies movement still exists today, held together by a small
    number of law professors, but it wields nowhere near the
    influence that the law and economics movement does when it

comes to actual public policy. See the Introduction to Posner, *Economic Analysis of Law*.

7 See generally G. S. Becker and J. J. Elias, "Introducing Incentives in the Market for Live and Cadaveric Organ Donation," *Journal of Economic Perspectives* 21(3):3–24, 2007, http://www.atypon-link. com/AEAP/doi/pdf/10.1257/jep.21.3.3.

8 David L. Kaserman and A. H. Barnett, *The U.S. Organ Procurement System: A Prescription for Reform* (Washington, DC: American Enterprise Institute Press, 2002), p. 134.

9 Kaserman, *The U.S. Organ Procurement System*, p. 52.

Chapter Six

1 See Organ Procurement and Transplantation Network, "Members: Regions," http://www.optn.org/members/regions.asp.

Chapter Seven

1 The Web site was originally found at www.kidney transplantations.com. However, that site is no longer in operation and its pages can no longer be found on the Internet. The domain name is now apparently owned by an unaffiliated entity. As discussed elsewhere, Dr. Shapira was subsequently arrested on charges of organ brokering in Turkey; he was released some weeks later, and rumors have since placed him in the Philippines, where the buying and selling of live kidneys is legal.

2 See Judy Siegel, "Surgeon Barred from Conducting Kidney Transplants," *Jerusalem Post* October 14, 1996; see also Michael Finkel, "This Little Kidney Went to Market," *New York Times* May 27, 2001, posted at http://web.mit.edu/writing/fee/2004_ FEE_July_Readin.htm; Nancy Scheper-Hughes, "The Global Traffic in Human Organs," *Current Anthropology* 41(2):191–224, 2000; Nancy Scheper-Hughes, "The Global Traffic in Human Organs: A Report Presented to the House Subcommittee on International Operations and Human Rights, United States Congress, June 27, 2001," http://www.publicanthropology.org/ TimesPast/Scheper-Hughes.htm.

3 See Scheper-Hughes, *Current Anthropology;* and Scheper-Hughes, House Subcommittee report. See also Finkel, "This Little Kidney Went to Market."

4 "An Israeli and an Arab Showing the Way," ArabicNews.com, May 15, 1998, www.arabicnews.com/ansub/Daily/Day/980513/1998051370.html.

5 See Finkel, "This Little Kidney Went to Market."

6 See generally Scheper-Hughes, House Subcommittee report; see also Nancy Scheper-Hughes, "Ends of the Body: The Global Commerce in Organs for Transplant Surgery," at http://sunsite.berkeley.edu/biotech/organswatch/pages/endsofbody.html; and Scheper-Hughes, *Current Anthropology.*

7 See Sheera Frenkel, "Organ-Trafficking Laws in Key Countries," *Christian Science Monitor* June 9, 2004, http://csmonitor.com/2004/0609/p12s02-wogi.html; Scheper-Hughes, House Subcommittee report; Scheper-Hughes, *Current Anthropology.*

8 Scheper-Hughes, *Current Anthropology.*

9 Larry Rohter, "The Organ Trade: A Global Black Market; Tracking the Sale of a Kidney on a Path of Poverty and Hope," *New York Times* May 23, 2004, http://www.nytimes.com/2004/05/23/international/americas/23BRAZ.html.

10 Abraham McLaughlin, Ilene R. Prusher, and Andrew Downie, "What Is a Kidney Worth?" *Christian Science Monitor* June 9, 2004, http://csmonitor.com/2004/0609/p01s03-wogi.html.

11 See Sheila M. Rothman and David J. Rothman, "The Organ Market," http://biology.franklincollege.edu/Bioweb/Biology/course_p/bioethics/Organ%20Market.doc.

12 Rothman, "The Organ Market."

13 "Pakistan, says an early August World Health Organisation report from Hong Kong, remains among the top five organ-trafficking hotspots besides China, Colombia, Egypt and the Philippines." Imtiaz Gul, "Inhumanity of Organ Trade," *The News International* August 13, 2007, posted at http://www.imtiazgul.com/24.html. The various WHO reports on the subject of the growing global markets for organs are invaluable. The most comprehensive is Y. Shimazono, "The State of the International Organ Trade:

A Provisional Picture Based on Integration of Available Information," *Bulletin of the World Health Organization* 85(12):901–980, 2007, http://www.who.int/bulletin/volumes/85/12/06-039370/en/index.html. Interestingly, despite all the pseudocoverage of the issue by observers ranging from Nancy Scheper-Hughes to David Kaserman, the Shimazono report bemoans the actual "paucity of scientific research." Compare generally D. Rothman, "International Organ Traffic," presented at the 10th Annual Conference on the Individual and the State, Central European University, Budapest, June 14–16, 2002, available in different form in the *New York Review of Books* 45(5), March 26, 1998.

14 Among the many is one titled "Welcome to One-Kidney Island," *ThirtySomething* v.4.3 December 5, 2007, http://writingthirty.blogspot.com/2007/12/welcome-to-one-kidney-island.html.

15 For a table that lists some of these Web sites based in China, Pakistan, and the Philippines, see Shimazono, "The State of the International Organ Trade." Web sites that are listed include http://www.liver4you.org and http://beverlyhills.ph (for the Beverly Hills Medical Group). And for one of the most lavish of the many Web sites that openly advertise for transplant tourism, see HealthToursIndia.com at http://www.healthtoursindia.com/transplant1.html.

16 Many pages of coverage on the issue appear on the Internet. The three that were relied upon most for the text were: Thomas Diflo, "Use of Organs from Executed Chinese Prisoners," *Lancet* 364:30–31, December 1, 2004; Craig S. Smith, "On Death Row: China's Source of Transplants," *New York Times* October 18, 2001, posted at http://www.crimlaw.org/defbrief169.html; and Shimazono, "The State of the International Organ Trade."

17 See generally the writings of Nancy Scheper-Hughes cited throughout "The Ends of the Body"; Scheper-Hughes, House Subcommittee report; and Scheper-Hughes, *Current Anthropology*. Many of these writings are repetitive and out-of-date, but Scheper-Hughes remains actively engaged in the fight against organ markets. She is a frequent speaker and prolific writer.

18 Again, volumes have been written about the organ trade in India. For this passage, the following were the most relied upon: Trupti Patel, "India Kidney Trade," *TED Case Studies* 5(1), January 1996,

http://www.american.edu/projects/mandala/TED/KIDNEY.
HTM; Ashwini R. Sehgal, "Sellers and Losers," *Frontline* 19(22),
October 26–November 8, 2002, http://www.hinduonnet.com/
fline/fl1922/stories/20021108004008100.htm, reporting on a
study conducted by Madhav Goyal, Ravindra L. Mehta, Law-
rence J. Schneiderman, and Ashwini R. Sehgal, "Economic and
Health Consequences of Selling a Kidney in India," *Journal of the
American Medical Association* 288(13):1589–1593, 2002; and G.
Ananthakrishnan, "Commerce in Kidneys on the Rise: Study,"
Hindu January 9, 2004, http://www.thehindu.com/2004/01/09/
stories/2004010904711200.htm. Also, Shimazono, "The State of
the International Organ Trade," and the collected works of
Nancy Scheper-Hughes provided additional detail and data, as
well as links and further references.

19 The incident was widely reported throughout the media. See
Karen Russo, "Indian Gang Accused of Stealing Human
Kidneys," ABC News, January 28, 2008, http://abcnews.go.com/
Health/story?id=4201900&page=1; "More Hospitals Linked to
Kidney Racket," AndhraCafe.com January 29, 2008, http://www.
andhracafe.com/index.php?m=show&id=31154; Amelia Gentleman, "Kidney Thefts Shock India," *New York Times* January 30,
2008, www.nytimes.com/2008/01/30/world/asia/30kidney.html;
Randeep Ramesh, "Britons Held in India Kidney Snatching
Investigation," *Guardian* January 31, 2008, http://www.guardian.
co.uk/world/2008/jan/31/india.randeepramesh1; Naleem Raaj,
"The Global Kidney Bazaar," *Times of India* February 3, 2008,
http://timesofindia.indiatimes.com/The_global_kidney_bazaar/
articleshow/2751820.cms; "Alleged Kidney Transplant Ring-
leader Arrested in Nepal," CBC News February 7, 2008, http://
www.cbc.ca/world/story/2008/02/07/amit-kumar.html; and
"Nepal Deports Transplant Suspect to India," CTV February 9,
2008, http://www.ctv.ca/servlet/an/local/CTVNews/
20080209/transplant_suspect_080209?hub=EdmontonHome.

20 Gentleman, "Kidney Thefts Shock India."

21 See generally Shimazono, "The State of the International Organ
Trade"; see also Zofeen Ebrahim, "Organ Transplant Law Won't
Stop Kidney Trade," Inter Press Service News Agency September
25, 2007, http://ipsnews.net/news.asp?idnews=39392: "Few in

Pakistan believe that a presidential ordinance, passed earlier this month, regulating organ transplantation will stop a flourishing but gruesome trade in human kidneys." In fact, several of the Pakistani Web sites that openly advertise for transplant tourists are listed in Shimazono, "The State of the International Organ Trade."

22 See Lubomyr Prytulak, "Israelis Deep into Organ Trafficking: Israel Asper, Letter 01, 10-May-2002, They Left Their Hearts in Tel Aviv," May 10, 2002, www.voicesofpalestine.org/outrageous/organtraffic.asp.

23 See generally Vidya Ram, "International Traffic in Human Organs," *Frontline* 19(7), March 30–April 12, 2002, http://www.hinduonnet.com/fline/fl1907/19070730.htm; see also Shimazono, "The State of the International Organ Trade." Live kidney sales are legal in Iran. The Charity Association for the Support of Kidney Patients and the Charity Foundation for Special Diseases are the nongovernmental organizations that facilitate the kidney trade; both are fully regulated by the strict Islamist government. See Frenkel, "Organ-Trafficking Laws in Key Countries."

24 Those who call for free capitalist markets in organs are a clamorous bunch. And the reality is simply that the "outright prohibition of organ sales . . . has not restricted the trade in [human body parts]; indeed, prohibition has tended to foster the trade, even as it has shaped the trade's emergence along traditional world economic lines." (Trevor Harrison, "Globalization and the Trade in Human Body Parts," *Canadian Review of Sociology and Anthropology* 36(1):21–35, 1999) However, the vast majority of countries in the world prohibit organ sales and the trend is against legalization, especially among Western cultures. See generally Patricia Marshall and Barbara Koenig, "Accounting for Culture in a Globalized Bioethics," *Journal of Law, Medicine and Ethics* 32(2):252–266, 2004. In particular, in June of 2003, the Social, Health and Family Affairs Committee of the European Parliament issued a report on trafficking in organs in Europe. At that time there were 120,000 patients on chronic dialysis and 40,000 waiting for kidneys in Western Europe alone. People were starting to buy and sell organs, and the problem was most acute in the Eastern European countries. The report called for the European Union to stop all trafficking in organs. See Parliamen-

tary Assembly, Council of Europe, "Trafficking in Organs in Europe," Recommendation 1611, June 25, 2003, http://assembly. coe.int/Documents/AdoptedText/TA03/EREC1611.htm; and Parliamentary Assembly, Council of Europe, "Trafficking in Organs in Europe," Document 9822, June 3, 2003, http://assembly. coe.int/Documents/WorkingDocs/Doc03/EDOC9822.htm. Four months later, the European Parliament approved tough new rules to curb organ trafficking. See European Parliament, "Prevention and Control of Trafficking in Human Organs," October 23, 2003, available online through http://europa.eu/documents; see also "Clampdown on Organ Transplant Tourism," October 28, 2003, a press release from the European Parliamentary Labour Party, available online under "Health and Disability" at http://www. erylmcnallymep.org.uk/pressrelease.htm.

25 See Shimazono, "The State of the International Organ Trade."

26 Stephen J. Dubner and Steven D. Levitt, "Flesh Trade: Weighing the Repugnance Factor," *New York Times Magazine* July 9, 2006, http://www.nytimes.com/2006/07/09/magazine/09wwln_freak. html; see also generally Gary S. Becker and Julio Jorge Elías, "Introducing Incentives in the Market for Live and Cadaveric Organ Donation," *Journal of Economic Perspectives* 21(3):3–24, 2007, http://www.atypon-link.com/AEAP/doi/pdf/10.1257/ jep.21.3.3.

27 Dubner, "Flesh Trade: Weighing the Repugnance Factor."

28 Dubner, "Flesh Trade: Weighing the Repugnance Factor."

29 Scheper-Hughes, *Current Anthropology;* see also Scheper-Hughes, House Subcommittee report.

30 Nancy Scheper-Hughes, "The Global Traffic in Human Organs," in Jonathan Xavier Inda and Renato Rosaldo, editors, *The Anthropology of Globalization: A Reader* (Malden, Massachusetts: Blackwell, 2002), pp. 270–308.

31 "Last night the Prime Minister threw his weight behind the campaign to change the system. . . . [I]n an interview with the Sunday Telegraph, Gordon Brown said: 'A system of this kind seems to have the potential to close the aching gap between the potential benefits of transplant surgery in the UK and the limits imposed by our current system of consent.' Ministers will embark

shortly on a review of the existing system." (Jo Revill and Deni Campbell, "Calls Grow for Organ Transplant Revolution," *Observer* January 13, 2008, http://www.guardian.co.uk/uk/2008/jan/13/politics.publicservices) Many European countries have adopted an "opt-out" or "presumed consent" system of organ recovery. Their relative track records in reducing their organ waiting lists, and the potential use of a presumed consent system to remedy the crisis in America's organ transplant policy, are discussed more fully in Chapters Eleven and Twelve.

Chapter Ten

1 For the Web site of the Transplantation Society, see http://www.transplantation-soc.org.

2 See generally Karen Auge, "Kidney Gift Is at Heart of Debate," *Denver Post* October 21, 2004, p. A-01 [editorial]; "Organ Donation Raises Legal, Ethical Concerns," *Denver Post* October 22, 2004, p. B-06; and "Kidney Recipient, Donor Doing Well," *Denver Post* October 22, 2004, p. B-02.

3 See Marsha Austin, "Activists Defend Private Deals to Match Organ Donor, Recipient," *Denver Post* October 26, 2004, posted at http://www.marylinstransplantpage.com/activists-defend04.htm.

4 See Auge, "Kidney Gift Is at Heart of Debate"; "Organ Donation Raises Legal, Ethical Concerns"; and "Kidney Recipient, Donor Doing Well."

5 See Marsha Austin and Chuck Plunkett, "Web Transplant Pact Sets Off Ethics Alarms: Medical Ethicists Condemn the Internet-Brokered Operation as Opening the Door to Fraud and Abuse and as Undermining a Time-Honored System," *Denver Post* October 24, 2004, p. A-01; and Marsha Austin and Chuck Plunkett, "Web Pact for Kidney Draws Fire," *Denver Post* October 24, 2004, p. A-01.

6 See generally Auge, "Kidney Gift Is at Heart of Debate"; "Organ Donation Raises Legal, Ethical Concerns"; and "Kidney Recipient, Donor Doing Well."

7 See George Merritt, "Kidney Donor Sought Redemption," *Denver Post* October 26, 2004, p. A-01; George Merritt, "Web Kidney Donor Is Jailed," *Denver Post* October 29, 2004, p. B-02.

8 Further information about the Technion–Israel Institute of Technology can be found on its Web site at http://www.technion. ac.il. On April 27, 2008, a press release from Technion boasted, "With publication of the final results of the European Union's research program for promising young scientists, the extent of the Technion's achievement has become apparent: The Technion places second among European universities and first in Israel, with seven of its young researchers receiving large research grants—more than 1 million Euro on the average per researcher. Among the universities represented is Cambridge in first place with nine winners."

9 See generally Thomas L. Friedman, *The World Is Flat: A Brief History of the 21st Century* (New York: Farrar, Straus and Giroux, 2005). Friedman's metaphor is brilliant, both intensely personal and vividly abstract. It's also catchy and accessible. For example, at p. 8: "The global competitive playing field was being leveled. The world was being flattened. . . . I was filled with both excitement and dread." And lest anyone forget the roots or basis of this so-called flattening phenomenon, Friedman repeatedly reminds us that it is plainly a function of globalization, which in turn is plainly a function of spreading market-based capitalism and its institutions.

10 Basic background information on Dr. Kam can be found on the Web site of the University of Colorado Health Sciences Center, http://www.uch.edu/about-our-doctors.

11 Karen Auge, "Organ Donors Form Own Line: Websites Lure Givers, Recipients; Critics Say Networks Hurt System," *Denver Post* January 20, 2004, p. B-01.

12 Bill Scanlon, "Surgeon Vows Not to Work with Internet Donors," *Rocky Mountain News* October 22, 2004; see also Bill Scanlon, "Transplant Called Off," *Rocky Mountain News* October 19, 2004; Bill Scanlon and Brian Cresente, "Transplant Back On," *Rocky Mountain News* October 20, 2004; and Bill Scanlon, "After Two-Day Delay, Procedure Appears a Success," *Rocky Mountain News* October 21, 2004.

13 Dr. Kam made this later statement during his interview with the authors, which is described more fully in Chapter 12.

14 Bill Scanlon, "Transplants Routine after Half-Century," *Rocky Mountain News* December 23, 2004.

15 Debra Melani, "Living Donors Offer New Hope to Liver Patients," *Rocky Mountain News* November 11, 2000, posted at http://www.marylinstransplantpage.com/donating00.htm.

16 Scanlon, "Transplants Routine after Half-Century."

17 See Steven Cojocaru, *Glamour, Interrupted: How I Became the Best-Dressed Patient in Hollywood* (New York: Collins, 2007).

Chapter Eleven

1 The reprint of NOTA in Appendix B includes these recent amendments to the *United States Code* 42, Section 274e, as quoted and discussed in the text.

2 See Denise Grady and Anahad O'Connor, "The Kidney Swap: Adventures in Saving Lives," *New York Times* October 5, 2004, http://www.nytimes.com/2004/10/05/health/05kidn.html.

3 See Patricia Sullivan, "Charles Norwood: Ga. Congressman Pushed for Patients' Bill of Rights," *Washington Post* February 14, 2007, http://www.washingtonpost.com/wp-dyn/content/article/2007/02/13/AR2007021300755.html; "Georgia Congressman Charlie Norwood Dies after Long Battle with Cancer," FoxNews.com February 13, 2007, www.foxnews.com/story/0,2933,251748,00.html; "Charlie Norwood," Sourcewatch.org, www.sourcewatch.org/index.php?title=Charlie_Norwood; and "Charlie Norwood," Wikipedia.com, http://en.wikipedia.org/wiki/Charlie_Norwood.

4 The bill was passed by the House on March 7, 2007, by a vote of 422 to zero and passed by the Senate by unanimous consent on July 9, 2007; it became law on December 21, 2007. See http://www.govtrack.us/congress/bill.xpd?bill=h110-710.

5 See NOTA, Section 274e, Subsection c, Paragraph 4, in Appendix B.

6 Carl Levin, "Senate Floor Statement on Living Kidney Organ Donation," July 9, 2007, http://levin.senate.gov/newsroom/release.cfm?id=278466.

7   See http://www.lifesharers.org.

8   See Adam J. Kolber, "A Matter of Priority: Transplanting Organs Preferentially to Registered Donors," *Rutgers Law Review* 55: 671–740, 2003, at 712. It is not unusual for articles in the nation's law journals to predict trends and upcoming changes in the legal environment. See, for example, Michael T. Morley, "Increasing the Supply of Organs for Transplantation Through Paired Organ Exchanges," *Yale Law and Policy Review* 21:221–262, 2003, at 223-224—published 4 years before the Charlie Norwood amendments to NOTA were passed.

9   See *Organ Donation and Recovery Improvement Act*, Public Law 108-216, 108th Congress, April 5, 2004, http://www.govtrack.us/congress/bill.xpd?bill=h108-3926.

10 See US Department of Health and Human Services, "Legislation and Legislative History," OrganDonor.gov, www.organdonor.gov/research/legislation.htm.

11 See United Network for Organ Sharing, "Allocation of Deceased Kidneys," http://www.unos.org/PoliciesandBylaws2/policies/pdfs/policy_7.pdf.

12 See United Network for Organ Sharing, "OPTN/UNOS Board Opposes Solicitation for Deceased Organ Donation," November 19, 2004, http://www.unos.org/news/newsDetail.asp?id=374 [press release].

13 See, for example, the four policy proposals issued by UNOS on July 13, 2007, and the additional proposal issued by UNOS on November 12, 2007. Downloadable files are available at http://www.unos.org/policiesAndBylaws/publicComment/proposalsArchive.asp.

14 See "Organ Donation Policies Under Review," broadcast January 7, 2008, with guests Michael Shapiro, vice chair of UNOS's ethics committee, and Robert Montgomery, chief of the transplant division at Johns Hopkins University and Hospital, available at http://minnesota.publicradio.org/display/web/2008/01/07/midmorning2.

15 See Section 2(h) of the UAGA of 1987, including the Prefatory Note and Comments, posted at http://www.law.upenn.edu/bll/archives/ulc/fnact99/uaga87.htm.

16 See *Colorado Revised Statutes* Section 12-34-103(6), 1998, repealed and replaced in its entirety by Colorado's enactment of the Revised UAGA, House Bill 07-1266, effective July 1, 2007.

17 See *Maine Statutes,* Title 22, Part 6, Chap. 710, Section 2911(2) ("Overriding donor intent").

18 Kevin Wack, "Organ Donor Law Gets First Test," *Portland Press Herald and Maine Sunday Telegram* December 15, 2004, http://pressherald.mainetoday.com/specialrpts/braindonors/041215brain.shtml.

19 The National Conference of Commissioners on Uniform State Laws has established a user-friendly Web site, http://www.anatomicalgiftact.org, which contains the full text of the Revised UAGA, as well as helpful links to information about the status of its enactment in the various states, significant endorsements, even PowerPoint presentations that summarize the changes to the statute. The prohibition against the buying and selling of organs appears in Section 16, whose operative language reads: "[A] person that for valuable consideration, knowingly purchases or sells a part for transplantation or therapy if removal of a part from an individual is intended to occur after the individual's death commits a [felony] and upon conviction is subject to a fine not exceeding [$50,000] or imprisonment not exceeding [five] years, or both." The Comments on Section 16 remind us that the Revised UAGA, like the first UAGA, applies only to postmortem donations: "This section applies only to anatomical gifts and is substantially the same as the provisions in the 1968 and 1987 Acts. It only applies to sales of parts intended to be recovered from a decedent after death for transplantation or therapy. It remains essentially unchanged from prior law. This section is consistent and in accord with the National Organ Transplant Act, 42 U.S.C. § 274(e)." Recall, in contrast, that NOTA's prohibition applies clearly, by the generality of its language, to both live donations and postmortem donations. See NOTA, Section 274e, in Appendix B.

20 See Revised UAGA, Section 8, "Preclusive Effect of Anatomical Gift, Amendment, or Revocation." Only time will tell whether the new statute accomplishes what the old statute did not, in terms of negating the family veto.

21 The tragic story of Terri Schiavo spawned an incredible media circus as well as an unusually detailed entry on the popular Web site Wikipedia: http://en.wikipedia.org/wiki/Terri_Schiavo.

22 A copy of this document was provided by Rose Medical Center in Denver, Colorado. At least 40 states and the District of Columbia are enrolled in the Five Wishes program. For more information on this program, see http://www.agingwithdignity.org/5wishes.html.

23 See Shelby E. Robinson, "Organs for Sale? An Analysis of Proposed Systems for Compensating Organ Providers," *University of Colorado Law Review* 70:1019–1050, 1999, p. 1022.

24 The law, known as the "Governor Robert P. Casey Memorial Organ and Tissue Donation Awareness Trust Fund," is codified at *Pennsylvania Consolidated Statutes* Title 20, Section 8622, adopted in 1994 and amended in 2000; see also generally Laurel R. Siegel, "Re-engineering the Laws of Organ Transplantation," *Emory Law Journal* 49(3):917–955, 2000, p. 941.

25 See D. Joralemon, "Shifting Ethics: Debating the Incentive Question in Organ Transplantation," *Journal of Medical Ethics* 27(1):30–35, 2001, quoted at http://jme.bmjjournals.com/cgi/content/full/27/1/30.

26 See Senate Bill 76, "Living Donor Tax Benefit to Cover Unreimbursed Expenses Related to Donation," reported at http://www.giftoflifemichigan.org/government/pending-legislation.htm.

27 See D. J. Perales, "Rethinking the Prohibition of Death Row Prisoners as Organ Donors: A Possible Lifeline to Those on Organ Donor Waiting Lists," *St. Mary's Law Journal* 34(3): 687–732, 2003; for additional proposals see also Robinson, "Organs for Sale?"

28 See Kevin Spence, "Bill Would Change Organ Donor System; Reduce Wait," *Cape Gazette* February 1, 2008, http://www.capegazette.com/storiescurrent/200802/organdonor020108.html.

29 See *State v. Powell*, 497 So. 2d 1188 (Fla. 1986), upholding Section 732.9185, *Florida Statutes* 1983; see also Kelly Ann Keller, "The Bed of Life: A Discussion of Organ Donation, Its Legal and Scientific History, and a Recommended 'Opt-Out' Solution to

Organ Scarcity," *Stetson Law Review* 32:855–895, 2003, posted at http://justice.law.stetson.edu/lawrev/abstracts/PDF/32-4Keller. pdf. Note that the Powell case dealt with an "opt-out" presumed consent law that applied to corneas, which are generally considered "tissues" versus "organs." Other legal commentators are not so quick to accept the opt-out system. See generally Alexander Powhida, "Forced Organ Donation: The Presumed Consent to Organ Donation Laws of the Various States and the United States Constitution," *Albany Law Journal of Science and Technology* 9(349):1–20, 1999.

30 See *Georgia Lions Eye Bank Inc. v. Lavant*, 255 Ga. 60, 335 S.E. 2d 127 (1985); certiorari denied 475 U.S. 1084, 1986.

31 See Kevin Spence, "Bill Would Change Organ Donor System; Reduce Wait."

32 See, e.g., Jo Revill and Denis Campbell, "Calls Grow for Organ Transplant Revolution," *Observer* January 13, 2008, http://www. guardian.co.uk/uk/2008/jan/13/politics.publicservices; "Support for Organ 'Presumed Consent,'" *Manchester Evening News* January 13, 2008, www.manchestereveningnews.co.uk/news/ health/s/1031806; and Hamish MacDonell, "Sturgeon Backs 'Presumed Consent,'" *Scotsman* January 13, 2008, http:// thescotsman.scotsman.com/latestnews/Sturgeon-backs-39 presumed-consent39-.3667988.jp; see previously Veronica English, "Is Presumed Consent the Answer to Organ Shortages? Yes," *British Medical Journal* 334:1088, 2007, www.bmj.com/ cgi/content/full/334/7603/1088.

33 Kieran Healy, "The Political Economy of Presumed Consent," posted at http://repositories.cdlib.org/uclasoc/trcsa/31. The quote is from the study's Abstract. Healy also says on page 5: "Advocates argue . . . that other countries have successfully implemented this kind of policy. . . . In fact, we know little about the empirical effects of presumed consent laws on procurement rates, or about cross-national variation in organ procurement more generally." She next sets forth a detailed table on page 6 that reveals something astonishing: *Most of the countries that have presumed consent also have some sort of family veto!* That means that, in order to adopt a European-style system in all of its facets, the United States

would likely have to undo its decades-long efforts, culminating in the Revised UAGA, to do away with the family veto.

34 Firat Bilgel, "Political Economy of Consent Legislation: A Panel Analysis of Cadaveric Donation." The quote is from the study's Abstract. This more complete statement appears on page 22:

> The empirical evidence presented herein confirms that countries in which presumed consent is enacted have 18-19% higher cadaveric donation rates on average, compared to informed consent countries, even if the presumed consent laws are not enforced. Results suggest that the magnitude of this effect is likely to help in alleviating the persistent organ shortage. Specifically, a wealthy, dominantly Catholic presumed consent country with greater civil liberties is more likely to have higher cadaveric donation rates, holding other factors constant. However, an increase in the potential pool of organs is more effective to combat organ shortage in wealthy informed consent countries and neither religious beliefs nor greater civil liberties play an effective role.

For even greater detail, see pages 15 to 17 and 19. With respect to the family veto, Bilgel specifically states on page 16: "First, this type of legislation does not, in theory, allow next of kin to override the donor's wish to donate. However, in most of the presumed consent countries, the next of kin can practically veto donation even if the decedent has previously revealed her preference to donate organs. The reason for considering the families' decision in the process has been to avoid public backlash and to comply with the individual's rights," citing Healy, "The Political Economy of Presumed Consent." In fact, much of the material in the Bilgel study duplicates material in the earlier Healy study.

35 See David Orentlicher, "Presumed Consent to Organ Donation: Its Rise and Fall in the United States," *Rutgers Law Review* 61 (forthcoming). The quote appears in the Abstract for the article, posted at http://papers.ssrn.com/sol3/papers.cfm?abstract_id=1207862.

36 Parts of this account of the pope's visit to Denver are adapted from George Weigel, *Witness to Hope: The Biography of Pope John*

Paul II (New York: Cliff Street Books, 1999), pp. 679–683. The quote from the pope appears on p. 683.

37 Nancy Scheper-Hughes, "The Global Traffic in Human Organs," *Current Anthropology* 41(2):191–224, 2000, pp. 19–22.

38 Scheper-Hughes, "The Global Traffic in Human Organs," p. 204.

39 Scheper-Hughes, "The Global Traffic in Human Organs," p. 206.

40 See G. J. Banks, "Legal and Ethical Safeguards: Protection of Society's Most Vulnerable Participants in a Commercialized Organ Transplantation System," *American Journal of Law and Medicine* 21:45–110, 1995, p. 107.

41 Banks, "Legal and Ethical Safeguards," pp. 83–97.

42 See Shaun D. Pattinson, "Paying Living Organ Providers," *Web Journal of Current Legal Issues* 2003, http://webjcli.ncl.ac.uk/2003/issue3/pattinson3.html.

Chapter Twelve

1 See Gary S. Becker and Julio Jorge Elías, "Introducing Incentives in the Market for Live and Cadaveric Organ Donations," http://home.uchicago.edu/~gbecker/MarketforLiveandCadaveric OrganDonations_Becker_Elias.pdf, at p. 1 (Abstract). The same article in slightly edited form, but without the Abstract, was published as Gary S. Becker and Julio Jorge Elías, "Introducing Incentives in the Market for Live and Cadaveric Organ Donation," *Journal of Economic Perspectives* 21(3):3–24, 2007, http://www.atypon-link.com/AEAP/doi/pdf/10.1257/jep.21.3.3. The page references in Notes 2–5 below refer to the later version that appears in the *Journal of Economic Perspectives*.

2 Becker, "Introducing Incentives," p. 10.

3 Becker, "Introducing Incentives," p. 12.

4 Becker, "Introducing Incentives," p. 16.

5 Becker, "Introducing Incentives," pp. 9–14, 21–22.

6 See Arthur J. Matas, "A Gift of Life Deserves Compensation: How to Increase Living Kidney Donation with Realistic Incentives," *Policy Analysis* (604):1–24, November 7, 2007, http://www.cato.org/pubs/pas/html/pa-604/pa-604index.html, p. 1.

7 Matas, "A Gift of Life," p. 1.

8 Matas, "A Gift of Life," p. 3.

9 Matas, "A Gift of Life," pp. 9, 14, 17.

10 Matas, "A Gift of Life," p. 19.

11 Matas, "A Gift of Life," pp. 4–5.

12 See NOTA, Section 274e(c)(2), Appendix B.

13 For general information about stem cells in a very accessible question-and-answer format, see http://www.mayoclinic.com/health/stem-cells/CA00081.

14 See T. M. S. Chang, "Artificial Cells, Blood Substitutes & Nanomedicine," www.medicine.mcgill.ca/artcell.

15 See "Opportunity—Graduate Students Interested in Research on Bioreactor Technology in Regenerative Medicine," www.mirm.pitt.edu/news/article.asp?qEmpID=30.

16 Information about state funding of stem cell research can be found on the Web sites of the Kaiser Family Foundation, http://www.statehealthfacts.org/comparetable.jsp?ind=112&cat=2, and the National Conference of State Legislatures, http://www.ncsl/programs/health/genetics/esstatefunds.htm.

17 Constance Holden, "Spotlight Shifts to Senate After Historic House Vote," *Science* 308(5727):1388–1389, June 3, 2005.

18 The saga of President Bush's first veto has been widely told. And Congresswoman DeGette has been persistent since then in pushing her stem cell legislation. The most basic search at her official Web site, http://degette.house.gov, reveals literally dozens of entries about her work on the issue, including a second successful legislative effort that ended in a second presidential veto. A recent article in the *Rocky Mountain News* describing her latest efforts included an excellent timeline of relevant legislative developments concerning stem cells. See M. E. Sprengelmeyer, "DeGette Back for Round 3

in Bid to Overturn Stem Cell Restrictions," *Rocky Mountain News*
May 8, 2008, http://www.rockymountainnews.com/news/2008/
May/08/degette-back-for-round-3-in-bid-to-overturn-stem. Here
is a synopsis of the timeline that appears in the article:
• August 9, 2001: President Bush places strict limits on
federally funded research on embryonic stem cells.
• July 18, 2006: Legislation to overturn Bush's limits passes
Congress.
• July 19, 2006: Bush issues his first-ever veto to block the
legislation.
• November 2006: Democrats regain control of Congress in
the midterm elections.
• April 11, 2007: Congress passes legislation to overturn Bush's
stem cell limits again.
• June 20, 2007: President Bush again vetoes the legislation.

19 Henry Fountain, "Does Science Trump All?" *New York Times*
May 29, 2005, http://www.nytimes.com/2005/05/29/
weekinreview/29foun.html [opinion].

20 Gina Kolata, "Name Games and the Science of Life," *New York
Times* May 29, 2005, http://www.nytimes.com/2005/05/29/
weekinreview/29kolata.html [opinion].

21 James Brooke, "Without Apology, Leaping Ahead in Cloning,"
New York Times May 31, 2005, http://www.nytimes.
com/2005/05/31/science/31kore.html.

22 Dr. Hwang's spectacular fall from grace was widely reported, and
it included allegations of both research and financial fraud. See
"S. Korea Scientist on Fraud Charge," BBC News May 12, 2006,
http://news.bbc.co.uk/2/hi/asia-pacific/4763973.stm ("The South
Korean cloning scientist who faked his stem cell research has
been charged with fraud and embezzlement").

23 See Coalition for Advancement of Medical Research, "National
Poll Shows Strong Support for Stem Cell and Therapeutic
Cloning Research," March 25, 2005, posted at http://www.
worldhealth.net/news/national_poll_shows_strong_support_for_
s [press release]. Depending on who is doing the polling, the

percentage of support ranges from roughly 65 to 75 percent. See Coalition for the Advancement of Medical Research, "Nearly Three-Quarters of America Supports Embryonic Stem Cell Research," May 16, 2006, www.camradvocacy.org/camr_news. cfm?rid=051606B [press release]. Additional poll results are available at the same site.

24 See Nicholas Wade, "Biologists Make Skin Cells Work Like Stem Cells," *New York Times* June 7, 2007, http://www.nytimes. com/2007/06/07/science/07cell.html; see also Brandon Keim, "Stem Cell Breakthrough Is Like 'Turning Lead into Gold,'" *Wired* November 20, 2007, http://www.wired.com/medtech/ stemcells/news/2007/11/skin_cell.

25 The quotes are from "Scientists Create Beating Heart," *Australian* January 14, 2008, http://www.theaustralian.news. com.au/story/0,25197,23048877-2703,00.html; see also "Beating Heart Created in Laboratory," *Medical News Today* January 14, 2008, http://www.medicalnewstoday.com/articles/93856.php; Sarah-Kate Templeton, "Hopes of Custom-Built Organs as Scientists Create Beating Heart," *Sunday Times* January 13, 2008, www.timesonline.co.uk/tol/news/uk/health/ article3177646.ece; and Julie Steenhuysen, "Beating Heart Created in Laboratory," Australian Broadcasting Corporation January 14, 2008, http://www.abc.net.au/science/articles/ 2008/01/14/2137790.htm.

26 The quotes are from Amanda Gardner, "New Therapies Could Change Organ Transplants," *U.S. News & World Report* January 23, 2008, http://health.usnews.com/usnews/health/ healthday/080123/new-therapies-could-change-organ- transplants.htm; see also Miranda Hitti, "Organ Transplant Without Lifelong Drugs," WebMD January 24, 2008, http:// www.webmd.com/news/20080124/organ-transplant-without- lifelong-drugs; and "Doctors Report Transplant Break- through," *Medical News Today* January 29, 2008, www.medical newstoday.com/articles/95443.php.

27 See "Woman Has First Face Transplant," BBC News November 30, 2005, http://news.bbc.co.uk/1/hi/health/4484728.stm. Since

first posting this historic story, BBC News has continued to cover it closely. Many additional follow-up pieces can be accessed easily at the same Web site.

28 See "Face Transplant Recipient 'Perfect,'" CBS News December 13, 2007, www.cbsnews.com/stories/2007/12/13/earlyshow/ health/main3614079.shtml.

29 The event was held on March 4, 2008, at Queen Elizabeth Hall, South Bank Arts Centre, London. The schedule for the event is posted at www.savingfaces.co.uk.

30 See Lawrence K. Altman, "First Face Transplant Performed in the U.S." *New York Times* December 16, 2008, http://www.nytimes.com/2008/12/17/health/17face.html; and Lawrence K. Altman, "First U.S. Face Transplant Described," *New York Times* December 17, 2008, http://www.nytimes.com/2008/12/18/health/s18face.html.

31 The language of modern commerce is seldom so blatant. For example, one advertisement for eggs simply says, "Egg Donors Needed to Give the Miracle of Life. . . . Help a Couple's Dream Come True." The purchase and sale of human eggs isn't mentioned in the advertisement; instead, it says, "All Donors receive $5,000 for their time and commitment." (*Denver Post* June 5, 2005, p. C3.); see also Center for Reproductive Medicine, "Financial Compensation," http://www.crmeggdonor.com/ compensation.html: "Donors are compensated $4,000 upon completion of their egg donation to their first couple. Many donors will donate a second and third time to other couples, and receive $4,000 for each additional donation."

Chapter Thirteen

1 See http://www.americantransplantfoundation.org.

2 See http://www.donoralliance.org.

3 The phrase comes from Larry Diamond's excellent article "The Democratic Rollback: The Resurgence of the Predatory State," *Foreign Affairs* March/April 2008, http://www.foreignaffairs.org/20080301faessay87204/larry-diamond/the-democratic-rollback.html.

Appendix A

1 Transplant Australia, http://www.transplant.org.au.

2 E. Cody, "Transplant-Tourism Cuts: China Tightens Rules on Providing Organs to Foreign Patients," *Wall Street Journal Asia* July 4, 2007.

3 Indian Holiday Pvt. Ltd., "Indian Govt. Laws for Human Organ Transplant," http://medicalindiatourism.com/medical-tourism/human-organs-transplant-laws-india.html.

4 Amelia Gentleman, "Kidney Thefts Shock India," *New York Times* January 30, 2008, http://www.nytimes.com/2008/01/30/world/asia/30kidney.html.

5 "India to Liberalize Organ Transplant Act and Launch Nationwide Awareness Campaign," Medindia.com January 27, 2008, http://www.medindia.net/news/India-to-Liberalize-Organ-Transplant-Act-and-Launch-Nationwide-Awareness-Campaign-32309-1.htm.

6 Yosuke Shimazono, "The State of the International Organ Trade: A Provisional Picture Based on Integration of Available Information," *Bulletin of the World Health Organization* 85(12):901–980, 2007.

7 Ahad J. Ghods, "Organ Transplantation in Iran," *Saudi Journal of Kidney Diseases and Transplantation* 18(4):648–655, 2007.

8 Japan Organ Transplant Network, http://www.jotnw.or.jp/english.

9 Sudeshna Sarkar, "The Global Kidney Bazaar," *ISN Security Watch* February 18, 2008, http://www.isn.ethz.ch/isn/Current-Affairs/Security-Watch/Detail/?id=54101&lng=en.

10 Saudi Center for Organ Transplantation, http://www.scot.org.sa.

11 "Saudi Arabia to Pay Non-Relatives $13,333 US for Donating Kidney," *Transplant News* December 2006.

12 Organización Nacional de Trasplantes (National Organization of Transplants), http://www.ont.es.

13 British Medical Association, "Organ Donation," November 27, 2008, http://www.bma.org.uk/health_promotion_ethics/organ_transplantation_donation/OrganDonation1108.jsp.

14 "PM Backs Automatic Organ Donation," BBC News January 13, 2008, http://news.bbc.co.uk/1/hi/health/7186007.stm.

15 Organ Procurement and Transplantation Network, http://www.optn.org.

ABOUT THE AUTHORS

S teve Farber is a founding partner and president of Brownstein Hyatt Farber Schreck, LLP, where he practices primarily business and corporate law, including acquisitions and mergers, and partnership and real estate matters. He received both his bachelor's degree and his Juris Doctor from the University of Colorado, and has practiced law in Denver ever since. Farber has played an integral role in shaping the city of Denver over the past several decades. He has represented parties in the development of many of Denver's major venues, including the Pepsi Center, where the Colorado Avalanche (NHL) and Denver Nuggets (NBA) play; INVESCO Field at Mile High, where the Denver Broncos (NFL) play; and the Denver Convention Center Hotel.

Actively involved in many political, charitable, and community causes, Farber sits on a number of boards, including the Anti-Defamation League, Children's Diabetes Foundation, Children's Hospital Foundation, and Denver Metro Chamber Foundation. Farber has received many awards and recognitions during his prestigious career, including the Del Hock Lifetime Achievement Award from the Metro Denver Chamber of Commerce (2004), the Distinguished Alumni Award for Private Practice from the University of Colorado School of Law (2007), and the Barbara Davis High Hopes Award in recognition of his many contributions to the community and to the Children's Diabetes Foundation (2007).

Farber served as cochairman for former governor Bill Owens's College for Colorado, and was invited by President William Jefferson Clinton to be a member of the Site Advisory Committee for the 2000 Democratic National Convention. Farber later would serve as the co-chair of the Host Committee for the 2008 Democratic National Convention. In 2008, he was named Businessperson of the Year by the *Rocky Mountain News* for his work in bringing the Democratic National Convention to Denver.

Harlan Abrahams is a lawyer, writer, and educator. In the 1970s, he earned his bachelor's degree and Juris Doctor from the University of Nebraska and, one year later, an advanced LLM degree from Harvard Law School. He began teaching law at age 24 and has taught at five law schools. He was the youngest professor, at age 29, to be granted tenure at his university. As a law professor, he taught many courses including Constitutional Law, Administrative Law, Intellectual Property, Jurisprudence, and Economic Regulation of the Competitive Process. Abrahams settled in Denver in 1982, where he has been a partner at two national law firms, specializing in corporate and securities law, the structuring of business entities, and mergers and acquisitions. Since the early 1990s, as a lecturer on public policy, he has focused on the relationships among economics, politics, and law, teaching courses on Globalization and Sovereignty, U.S. Relations with Cuba, and the Regulatory Process.

Abrahams has published many scholarly articles on law and public policy. One of his novels has been optioned for a movie to be shot on location in Havana. He lives with his wife, Carolyn, and is currently writing his next book, about the changes happening in Cuba under Raúl Castro. He began following, researching, and writing about the global markets for human transplant organs more than 20 years ago.

INDEX

Boldface page references indicate photographs.
<u>Underscored</u> references indicate charts.

Abrams, Rick, 35–36, 97
Allocation of organs, 8–9, 42–43, 61, 69–71, 156–57
Alpert, Debbie, 103
Alpert, Lee, 51, 103
Alvarez, Steve, 4
American Society of Transplant Surgeons, 143
American Transplant Foundation, 201
Amnesty International, 114
Anita (nurse), 113
Antisodomy law, 30
Artificial organs research, 193
Asper, Israel, 90
Avila, José, 138, 141

Band-Aid approach, 157, 169, 175, 188
Banks, Gloria, 174–75
Barnard, Christian, 11
Barnett, A. H., 55–57
Becker, Gary S., 188–89
Black market organ trade and trafficking, 10–11, 76–86, 93–94
Bodily integrity issue, 28–31, 167
Boyles, Peter, 21
Bradley, Bill, 20
"Brain death" concept, 43
Brazil, 84, 93–94
Brown, Gordon, 94, 166
Brown, Hank, 69
Brownstein, Norm, 20–21, 37, 62, 68, 120, 124, 131
Brownstein, Sunny, 120, 131
Buddhism, 43
Burn treatments, 17–18, 137
Bush, George W., 152, 156, 193, 195, 206

Cadaveric organ donations, 9, 43–44, 69
Cadaveric organ sales, 55–57
Calne, Sir Roy, 18, 137
CanWest Global Communications Corporation, 90
Capitalism, 9–12, 205

Carolyn (business partner of Jim Sullivan), 101–2, 125
Castle, Mike, 194
Catholicism, 43, 167, 171
Cell transplants, 140. *See also* Stem cell research
Chan, Laurence "Larry," 130, 134–41, 163, 193
Charlie W. Norwood Living Donation Act, 40, 151–55, 157, 224–39
Children's Hospital (Denver), 14–15, 20
China, 86–87, 90, 185, 199, 205, <u>218–19</u>
Christianity, 43
Christian Science Monitor article on organ trade, 84–85
Citizen Kane (film), 73–74
Class issues. *See* Poor and market for organ transplants
Clinton, Bill, 21, 111, 130, 172
Clinton Library fundraiser, 21, 111, 130–31
Cloning, therapeutic, 195–96
CNN video on organ trade, 89
Cohen, Rabbi, 119–20
Cojocaru, Steven, 147–48, 203
Colombia, 90, 185
Commodification of body parts, 44, 94–95, 173, 175–76
Compensation for organ donations, 186–92, 206, 214
Consent laws, 40
Cook, Herb, 37–38, 116, 121, 123
Cosmas, St., 18–19
Coumadin, 135–36
Creatine, 36
Crosby, David, 201–2
Cuba, 205
Cyclosporine, 18–19

Damian, St., 18–19
Daniel, Moshe, 181–82
Davis, Marvin and Nancy, 146–47
DeGette, Diana, 194
Delaroca, Edgar, 7, 23, 25–26, 47, 50, 114, 207

Delaroca, Ernesto. *See also* Delaroca,
  Sandra
    Anita (nurse) and, 113
    aunt and, 7, 23–25, 27
    brother and, 7, 23, 25–26, 47, 50, 114,
      207
    California vacation and, 207
    Carolyn and, 102
    childhood of, 4–5, 7–8, 23–24
    cousin and, 24
    daughter and, 47, 114–15, 207–8, **211**
    disadvantages facing, 141
    emigration of, 24–25, 112
    Farber (Gregg) and, 209
    Farber (Steve) and, 209–10, **211**
    in Guatemala, 4–5, 7–8, 23, 179–80
    legalization as US citizen, 26–27
    nephews and, 50, 207–8, **211**
    parents and, 4–5, 7–8, 23
    in present time, 148, 209
    reunion with Farber family and, 207–10
    shortage of transplant organs and,
      8, 13
    sister and, 3–4, 23, 25–28, 46–47
    son and, 213
    Sullivan (Jim) and, 101–3
    Sullivan (Lynne) and, 121, 123
    transplant surgery of sister and
      convergence with Farber family
        and, 3–4
      day of, 114–15, 123–24, 126
      days after, 141
      decision about, 48–51
      eight months after, 146–48
      first anniversary of, 177–79
    uncle and, 23, 27
    wife and, 25–27, 48, 50, 114, 177, 207,
      211
Delaroca, Ernesto Angel, 213
Delaroca, Galilea "Gali," 47, 114–15,
  207–8, **211**
Delaroca, Gicela, 25–27, 48, 50, 114, 177,
  207–8, **211**
Delaroca, Rosalea, 4–5, 7–8, 23
Delaroca, Sandra
    brother Edgar and, 7, 23, 25–26, 47
    brother Ernesto and, 3–4, 23, 25–28,
      46–47
    childhood of, 23
    dialysis and, 28, 47–48, 50
    disadvantages facing, 141
    emigration of, 25
    in Guatemala, 23, 46
    kidney problem of, 27–28, 46–47
    legalization as US citizen, 26–27

    parents of, 4–5, 7–8, 23
    in present time, 148
    sister-in-law and, 48
    transplant surgery of
      convergence with Farber family
        and, 3–4
      day of, 113–14, 123–24, 126
      days after, 141
      decision about, 48–51
      first anniversary of, 177–79
    on waiting list, 28, 46
Delaroca, Valentine, 4–5, 7–8, 23
Delaware, 165–66, 169
Delmonico, Francis, 165
Denver Chamber of Commerce, 131–32
Dialysis, 28, 37, 47–48, 50, 117
Diflo, Thomas, 86
Doerflinger, Richard, 196

E gypt, 90
Elías, Julio Jorge, 188–89
Engelhardt, H. T. Jr., 44
Engleberg, David, 133–34
Ethical issues, 44–45, 51–53, 106
Europe, 93–94
European Union, 206

F *ace/Off* (film), 198
Face transplant, 198–200
Facial Surgery Research
  Foundation, 199
Family veto of organ donations, 159–61,
  167
Farber, Andie, 118, 208–9, **212**
Farber, Brad, 75, 97–98, **111**, 118, 121,
  157–60
Farber, Brent, 75, 97–99, 105, **111**, 118,
  121, 134
Farber, Cindy. *See also* Farber, Steve, wife
  and
    brother-in-law and, 96–97, 107
    granddaughter and, **212**
    mother's cancer and, 16–17
    National Kidney Foundation event
      and, 34–35
    reunion with Delaroca family and,
      208
    sister and, 107, 109
    son Brad and, 159
    son Gregg and, 4, 70, 105, **212**
    Sullivan (Jim) and, 99
    Sullivan (Lynne) and, 39, 65–68

Farber, Cindy. *See also* Farber, Steve, wife and (cont.)
  trips of
    Hawaii, **111**, 146–47
    Italy, 64, 68
    Mexico, 109
    Vienna, 169
    Warsaw, 169–70
Farber, Gregg, 3–4, 70, 75, 96–99, 104–12, **111**, 118–20, 128–29, 132, 204–5, 208–9, **212**
Farber, Janet, 14–15
Farber, Nathan, 14–15
Farber, Steve
  award bestowed on, 131–32
  brother-in-law and, 51, 77
  career of, building, 19–22
  Carolyn and, 101–2
  Chan and, 134–40
  childhood of, 14–17, 19–20
  Cojocaru and, 147–48
  coworkers and illness of, 62–63
  decisions facing, gut-wrenching, 71–75, 95–96
  Delaroca (Ernesto) and, 209–10, **211**
  donors for, possible, 70–71, 95
  father-in-law and, 37–38, 116
  Fox News interview and, 202–5
  granddaughter and, 118, 208–9, **212**
  at Johns Hopkins Hospital, 36–37, 39, 67–68
  kidney problems of, 14–17, 35–37, 158, 201
  Klug and, 202–3
  "measles cure" and, 14–17, 35
  mother-in-law's cancer and, 16–17
  National Kidney Foundation event and, 34–35
  nephrologist's advice to, 103–4
  nightmare of, 214–15
  parents of, 14–15
  as power broker, 21–22, 34–35
  purpose in life and, 201–2
  reflections of, 215
  reunion with Delaroca family and, 207–10
  Sara and, 104
  shortage of transplant organs and, 8, 13
  son Brad and, 75, 97–98, **111**, 157–60
  son Brent and, 75, 97–99, 105, **111**, 134
  son Gregg and, 3–4, 70, 75, 96–99, 104–12, **111**, 118–20, 128–29, 132, 204–5, 208–9
  Sullivan (Jim) and, 37–39, 51, 99–101

    Sullivan (Lynne) and, 51, 65, 67, 80–81, 85–86
  transplant surgery of
    convergence with Delaroca family and, 3–4
    day of, 3, 115, 120–21, 127
    days after, 127–30
    drug treatments, 128–29, 135
    first anniversary of, 169, 177
    return to public life after, 130–32
    son Gregg as donor for, 3, 70
    two days before, 119–20
  trips of
    Hawaii, **111**
    Italy, 64, 68
    Mexico, 107–12
    Prague, 170, 177
    Vienna, 169–72
    Warsaw, 169–70
  Turkey option and, 76–83
  on waiting list, 61–63, 68
  wife and
    award bestowed on husband, 131–32
    day of husband's surgery, 120–22, 124, 127
    illness of husband, 51
    Johns Hopkins Hospital visit, 37, 39
    options for husband's transplant surgery, 74–75, 77, 96–97, 99, 115–16, 118–19, 161
    recovery of husband, 131
    two days before husband's surgery, 119
Fetishization of life concept, 41
Fifth Amendment to US Constitution, 30
Finnegan, Cole, 110
First Amendment to US Constitution, 29–30
"Five Wishes" document, 162–63
Florida, 69, 166
Foster, Steven, 116
Fourth Amendment to US Constitution, 30
France, 199
Free exercise clause (First Amendment to the US Constitution), 29
Free Market Camp, 11, 51, 53–57, 180, 187, 191
Friedlaender, Michael, 83
Friedman, Milton, 55
Friedman, Thomas L., 32, 205

Garcia, Richard, 26–27
Garwood-Gowers, Austin, 29
Globalization, 9–12, 32–33, 205–6

Great Britain, 166, _222–23_
Guatemala, 4–8, 23, 46, 84, 179–80

Hansmann, Henry B., 54
Harrison (nephew of Ernesto Delaroca), 207–8, **211**
Healy, Kieran, 166–67
Heart, creating beating, 196–97
Heart transplant, 19
Hickenlooper, John, 130
Hickey, Bob, 142–43, 145, 192
Hinduism, 44
Human organ paired donation, 40, 151–55, 163–64, 189
Human Rights Camp, 11, 51–52, 54–55, 57, 180, 187, 191
Human Tissue Act (1983), 84
Husted, Bill, 131
Hwang, Woo Suk, 194–95
Hyatt, Jack, 20–21

Immunosuppressant drugs, 18–19, 135, 137, 147, 197–98
India, 10, 53, 56, 87–90, _218–19_
Informed consent, 29
Integrity of the body issue, 28–31, 167
International Kidney Exchange, 87
International Monetary Fund, 12, 205
Internet and organ donations, 142–43, 145
Iran, 10, 56, 91, _218–19_
Islam, 43
Island, The (film), 208
Israel, 81–82, 90–91, 183–85
Italy, 167

Jacobs, H. Barry, 87
Japan, _220–21_
Jewish people during World War II, 169–71
John Paul II, 43, 172–73
Johns Hopkins Hospital, 36–37, 39, 67–68
Jones, Jim, 109–10
José (uncle of Ernesto Delaroca), 23, 27
Judaism, 43, 119
Justinian, 18–19

Kam, Igal, 79, 113, 116–18, 130, 136, 140, 143–46, 161, 180–87, 192
Kaserman, David L., 55–57

Kidney disease and transplants, 85, 93, 142. _See also_ Delaroca, Sandra; Farber, Steve
Klein, Mel, 36, 61
Klug, Chris, 202–3
Kortz, Don, 131
Kumar, Amit "Dr. Horror," 89

Lamm, Richard D., 42
Latin America, 84–85, 93–94, 205
Laws, organ transplant, 40, 69, 87, _218–23_. _See also specific country and law_
Legal issues, 28–29, 106
Levin, Carl, 153–54
Lieberman, Joe, 35
Life insurance, 92
LifeSharers.com, 145, 155
Linkow, Mark, 97
Liver transplant, 19, 69, 145–46, 202–3
Lung transplant, 19
Lustig, Debbie, 107, 109, 120–23
Lustig, Jimmy, 51, 77, 96–97, 107, 120–21, 123

MacMillan, Bill and Deb, 34–35
Mantle, Mickey, 69
Marcos, Ferdinand, 85
Market for organs. _See also specific country_
  black, 10–11, 76–86, 93–94
  capitalism and, 9–12, 205
  class issues and, 88–89, 95
  commodification of body parts and, 44, 94–95, 173, 175–76
  foreign, 10, 83–84
  free, possibility of adopting, 165–66, 173–75
  Free Market Camp and, 11, 51, 53–57, 180, 187, 191
  globalization and, 9–12, 32–33, 205–6
  growth of, 33, 83–84
  Human Rights Camp and, 11, 51–52, 54–55, 57, 180, 187, 191
  organ donations and, 185
  poor and, 53, 56, 81, 88–89
  pros and cons of, 51–57
  regulation of, proposed, 174–75
  Scheper-Hughes and, 51–53, 82, 84, 87–88
  sovereignty issue and, 11–12, 31–32, 206
  stealing organs and, 84
  volunteer, 93
Marx, Karl, 41
Matas, Arthur, 189–92

MatchingDonors.com, 142–43, 145
Mayo Clinic, 14–17
McDonald, Kirk, 132
McIndoe, Sir Archibald, 17
"Measles cure," 14–17, 35
Medawar, Peter, 17–18
Medical tourism, 56, 85, 92
Metzger, Robert, 156
Michigan, 165
Morgan, Tara, 61, 159
Morris, Sir Peter, 137
Murray, Joseph, 19

National Kidney and Transplant
    Institute (Philippines), 85
National Kidney Foundation event, 34–35
National Organ Transplant Act (NOTA)
    ban on cadaveric organ sales and,
        55–56
    Charlie W. Norwood Living Dona-
        tion Act and, 40, 151–55, 157,
        224–39
    human organ paired donation and,
        151–55, 163–64, 189
    implementation of, 40
    operation of Organ Procurement and
        Transplantation Network and, 40
Nepal, 89
New York Times investigation of organ
    trade, 84
Norwood, Charlie, 152
NOTA. See National Organ Transplant
    Act

Obama, Barack, 141, 192, 206, 213
One-Kidney Island (Manila), 86
"Opt-in" system, 40, 165
OPTN, 9, 40, 43, 70–71
"Opt-out" system, 40, 94, 165–69, 173,
    188
Orentlicher, David, 168
Organ Donation and Recovery Improve-
    ment Act, 156
Organ Donation Awareness Trust Fund,
    164–65
Organ donations
    Band-Aid approach and, 157, 169,
        175, 188
    Chan's vision of, 140–41
    Charlie W. Norwood Living Dona-
        tion Act and, 40, 151–55, 157,
        224–39

compensation for, 186–92, 206, 214
consent laws and, 40
family discussions about, lack of,
    161–62
family veto and, 159–61, 167
human organ paired, 40, 151–55,
    163–64, 189
through Internet, 142–43, 145
Kam's view of, 145, 185–86
lack of, 39
lawsuits involving wrongful taking of
    organs and, 160
market for organs and, 185
Matas's view of, 189–91
in Michigan, 165
organ donation forms and, 163
in Pennsylvania, 164–65
postmortem/cadaveric, 9, 43–44, 69
presumed consent system and, 40, 94,
    165–69, 173, 188
tests needed before, 163
Organ failure, 148
Organ Procurement and Transplantation
    Network (OPTN), 9, 40, 43, 70–71
Organs Watch, 40–41, 82, 84
Organ transplants. See also Delaroca,
    Sandra; Farber, Steve; specific country;
    Transplant surgery; Waiting list for
    organ transplants
    bodily integrity issue and, 28–31, 167
    Chan's vision of, 140
    commodification of body parts and,
        44, 94–95, 173, 175–76
    Delaroca-Farber families and, 3–4,
        214–15
    ethical issues and, 44–45, 51–53, 106
    fetishization of life concept and, 41
    informed consent and, 29
    legal issues of, 28–29, 106
    privacy rights and, 29–30, 168
    reform of, need for, 214
    religion and, 43–44
    resources and information about,
        39–40
    Scheper-Hughes and, 40–42, 174
    skin cells for, research on, 195–96
    sovereignty issue and, 11–12, 31–32,
        206
    stem cell research and, 193, 206
    supply-and-demand gap and, 93, 164
Ortiz, Louise, 28
Oswaldo (cousin of Ernesto Delaroca), 24
Otilia (aunt of Ernesto Delaroca), 7,
    23–25, 27
Ott, Harold, 197

Pakistan, 10, 91, 185
Parker, Penny, 131
Pattinson, Shaun, 175
Peña, Federico, 109–10
Pennsylvania, 164–65
Peri, Ilan, 84
Philippines, 10, 85–86, 90–91, 185, 205, 220–21
Phylacteries, 119
Poor and market for organ transplants, 53, 56, 81, 88–89, 95
Posner, Richard, 55
Postmortem organ donations, 9, 43–44, 69
Postmortem organ sales, 55–57
Prednisone, 129
Presumed consent system, 40, 94, 165–69, 173, 188
Privacy rights, 29–30, 168
Puche, Jamie Serra, 109

Raul (nephew of Ernesto Delaroca), 50
Reagan administration, 5
Reform of organ transplant system, need for, 13, 214
Religion, 43–44
Revised UAGA, 163–64, 167–69
Ricketson, Mary, 130–31
Rios Montt, José Efrain, 5–6
Robinson, Mitch, 120
Roe v. Wade, 30
Romer, Roy, 172

Salazar, Ken, 130
Sapkin, Rick and Shelley, 123
Sara (wife of Gregg Farber), 75, 104, 118–19, 125, 129
Satz, Debra, 10, 53–54
Saudi Arabia, 220–21
Scadden, David, 196
Scheper-Hughes, Nancy, 40–42, 51–53, 82, 84, 87–88, 174
Schiavo, Terri, 162–63
Schlenker, Sidney, 38, 66
Schwartzkopf, Pete, 166
Sewal, Sarah "Hospital Sarah," 120–21, 123, 125
Shanahan, Mike, 115
Shapira, Zaki, 76–83, 90–92, 97, 105, 137, 151–52, 183–85, 187, 205, 213–14

Shinto, 44
Shore, Jim, 68–69
Shortage of transplant organs, 8–9, 13, 39, 93, 164
Silva, Alberty José da, 84
Skin cells for organ transplants, research on, 195–96
Skin grafting, 17–18, 137
Smitty, Samuel Robert, 142–45, 192
Smythe, W. Roy, 197
Sol (fictitious name), 76–77
Somatic cell nuclear transfer, 194
South Africa, 10, 84–85, 174
South Korea, 194
Sovereignty issue, 11–12, 31–32, 206
Spain, 167, 220–21
Starzl, Thomas, 19, 145–46
Stem cell research, 140, 192–97, 206, 214
Stem Cell Research Enhancement Act, 194–95
Sullivan, Jim, 37–39, 51, 64–66, 68, 99–103, 124, 208
Sullivan, Lynne, 37, 39, 51, 64–68, 80–81, 85–86, 114, 120–25, 208
Supply-and-demand gap in organ transplants, 93, 164

Taylor, Doris, 196–97
Technion-Israel Institute of Technology, 144
Tefillin, 119
Tendler, Moses, 43
Thailand, 85
Therapeutic cloning, 195–96
Transplantation Society, 138
Transplant surgery. See also Delaroca, Sandra; Farber, Steve
    complications after, 53
    face, 198–200
    heart, 19
    historical perspective, 17–19
    liver, 19, 69, 145–46, 202–3
    lung, 19
    modern era of, 19
    organ failure and, 148
    skin grafting, 17–18
    success stories, 203
    tranformative effects of, 202
Transplant tourism, 56, 85, 92
Tuchman, Ken, 77
Turkey, 10, 77–83, 90–91
Turner, Shaul, 203–5

Uniform Anatomical Gift Act
(UAGA), 40, 70, 159–61, 163–64,
167–69
United Kingdom, 166, <u>222–23</u>
United Nations, 12, 32, 206
United Network for Organ Sharing
(UNOS), 9, 40, 143, 155–57
United States
   allocation of organs in, 8–9, 42–43,
     69–71
   Charlie W. Norwood Living Organ
     Donation Act and, 40, 151–55, 157,
     224–39
   "Five Wishes" document and, 162–63
   flawed organ transplant policy of, 148
   free market for organ transplants and,
     possibility of adopting, 165–66,
     173–75
   health care system and reform in,
     141–42
   kidney transplants in, 93
   market for organs in, 8–9, 93
   "opt-in" system in, 165
   options for organ transplants in,
     92–93
   Organ Donation and Recovery
     Improvement Act and, 156
   Organ Donation Awareness Trust
     Fund and, 164–65
   organ transplant laws in, <u>222–23</u>
   presumed consent system and, pos-
     sible, 94, 167–69
   reform of organ transplant system in,
     13, 214
   regional basis of Organ Procurement
     and Transplant Network and,
     70–71
   shortage of transplant organs in, 8–9,
     13, 39, 93, 164
   state differences in waiting lists in, 69
   supply-and-demand gap in organs
     and, 93

volunteer market for organs in, 93
University of Chicago, 55
University of Colorado Health Sciences
   Center, 116, 145, 201
University of Colorado Hospital, 49, 202
University of Minnesota, 196
UNOS, 9, 40, 143, 155–57
US constitutional law, 28–31, 206
US Department of Health and Human
   Services, 40, 43
US Supreme Court, 29–30, 166, 168, 206

Victores, Oscar Humberto Mejía, 6
Voice of Palestine Web site, 90
Volunteer market for organs, 93

Waiting list for organ transplants
   cadaveric organs and, 69
   Delaroca (Sandra) on, 28, 46
   Farber (Steve) on, 61–63, 68
   Human Rights Camp and, 54
   rise in, 93
   state differences in, 69
   statisticss on, 9, 42
   United Network for Organ Sharing
     and, 9, 155
Webb, Wellington and Wilma, 130
WHO, 86, 90, 92
Wirth, Tim, 109–10
World Bank, 205
World Health Organization (WHO), 86,
   90, 92
World Trade Organization, 12, 205–6
World War II, 17, 32, 137, 169–71

Yamanaka, Shinya, 196